*Why David Hated Tuesdays*

# Why David Hated Tuesdays

## *One Courageous Mother's Guide to Keeping Your Family Toxin and Allergy Free*

Amilya Antonetti

PRIMA PUBLISHING

Published by Prima Publishing, Roseville, California. Member of the Crown Publishing Group, a division of Random House, Inc.

PRIMA PUBLISHING and colophon are trademarks of Random House, Inc., registered with the United States Patent and Trademark Office.

**Library of Congress Cataloging-in-Publication Data**
Antonetti, Amilya.
    Why David hated Tuesdays : one courageous mother's guide to keeping your family toxin and allergy free / Amilya Antonetti.— 1st ed.
        p. ; cm.
    Includes bibliographical references and index.
    ISBN 0-7615-1499-6
    1. Housing and health—Popular works.  2. Detoxification (Health).
3. Multiple chemical sensitivity—Popular works.
[DNLM: 1. Multiple Chemical Sensitivity—prevention & control—
Child—Personal Narratives.  2. Multiple Chemical Sensitivity—
prevention & control—Child—Popular Works. WA 30.5 A634w 2003]
I. Title.
RA770 .A56 2003
616.97—dc21
2002155838

    05  06  TT  10  9  8  7  6  5  4  3  2
Printed in the United States of America

First Edition

**Visit us online at www.primapublishing.com**

*Life is full of great blessings, and my son, David, is one of mine.*

■   ■   ■

This book is dedicated to you, David, my greatest success.
You make my life more complete, and I thank God for you
every day. May I help guide you on your journey through life
and encourage you to spread your wings and fly.

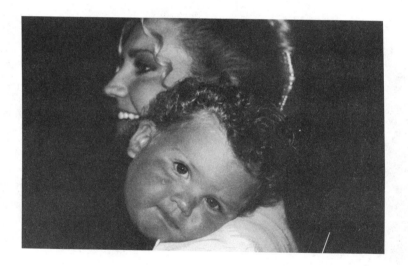

# Contents

# Acknowledgments

When I find myself fading, I close my eyes and realize my friends
are my energy.
—Anonymous

OUR JOURNEY THROUGH LIFE is built of many tiny steps, some easy and others that threaten to break us in two. Each step has shaped me into who I am. Writing this book showed me how many wonderful people have shared those steps with me. I am very blessed to have these and so many others in my life.

My parents, Bette ann and Franco Antonetti, each gave a piece of who they were, which made me who I am today. Sadly, my mother passed on when I was young. Her gifts to me were her creativity, humor, and zest for life. My respect for hard work, my commitment to myself and others, and the force that moves me through life with determination, strength, and tenacity all come from my father. My father, who got off the boat from Italy as a young man, deeply ingrained in me his love for this country and for the people who built it and encouraged me to embrace the opportunities that I am so lucky to have.

My brother, "Buddy," has laughed and cried with me every step of life's journey. I am so proud of the man he has become. He continues to add so much to my life. Thank you!

My childhood girlfriend and still best friend, Carol Klepacz-Dashiell, showers me with unconditional support and forces me to keep myself grounded. She helps me be a better person. My girlfriends Robin Gomes and Sheila Lightner keep me laughing at myself and at life. My colleagues, Young Entrepreneurs Organization friends, and other entrepreneurs along the way have encouraged me and taught me the ins and outs of business; I am truly grateful to them all.

Without the belief and support of Annette Davidson from Trader Joe's, I would not be before you in business today. She patiently taught me, believed in me, and encouraged me to keep going. I don't have the words to tell you what that means to me. Thank you!

My ex-husband and David's father, Dennis Karp, continues to be an integral part of my life. I am grateful for the time we shared and continue to share together. The love we have for each other and for our son is a true blessing. We continue to support each other in our separateness and focus on building a solid foundation for our son.

Jeff and Merrie Wycoff touch me in so many ways that my life will never be the same. Thank you for your belief in me. Thank you for your love of Soapworks. My gratitude can never be measured. I will love you both forever.

This book would never have been written without the hard work, love, and encouragement of Katherine Sansone. God sent me an angel the day we met. Thank you for sharing your knowledge, wisdom, humor, and yourself with me and this book.

My life changed forever when my path crossed that of Anthony Tesoriero. His love fills me to the point of overflow, his belief in me brings me to tears, his wisdom and knowledge push me to learn more. His spirit lifts me to new levels. I love you.

And finally, to everyone along the way who has given a part of yourself to my son and me, thank you!

# Preface

A journey of a thousand miles must begin with a single step.
—Lao-tzu (604–531 B.C.), *The Way of Lao-tzu*

HOW MANY TIMES do we go outside ourselves to find the answer to a problem? I spent so much time when my son, David, was ill thinking that someone else knew more about my life and its challenges than I did. I spent a great deal of time sitting through seminars and reading self-help books in search of answers to questions about life balance, career, and fulfillment. We are taught to look to "experts" for our answers, only to find out that they often have no real-life experience on the subject. When all is said and done, change begins with you. Strength, willpower, responsibility, commitment, and integrity grow from within and blossom only under your direction.

Many of today's women are CEOs, managers in all types of industries, and entrepreneurs, yet we are still the foundation of our families. In the home, we are a friend, lover, cook, housekeeper, taxi driver, and the "do for me, get for me" person. I was no exception.

When David was born, nine years ago, I added a new title to my list—parent. Because I was parenting a sick baby, however, my list of titles extended further: I became an expert at understanding medical terms, conditions, and treatments so that I could speak to the doctors and nurses intelligently. I became an at-home chemist, cooking up soaps in my kitchen. I became a researcher, investigating, writing letters, and making inquiries to environmental organizations and alternative health practitioners. I began corresponding and working with consumer advocates who could help me understand what was causing my son's illnesses. In short, the skills and determination that made me a successful businessperson were now helping me learn how to free my son from the toxins that were destroying him.

I think it is not only my anger but also my guilt that drives me on my quest to inform others about chemicals and toxins and their potential harm. Even now, nearly a decade after David's birth, I carry the guilt of a single question—"Why didn't I know?" Why didn't I know what was causing David's horrifying sickness? After all, hadn't I taken parenting classes and read everything I could get my hands on while pregnant? Despite my preparation for his birth, I was still absolutely clueless about the dangers that faced him in the home. Why did it take almost two years of my son's life to figure out what was causing his illness and begin turning his life around into a healthy one by making changes to our home and lifestyle? And if I was a mom who was reading and looking for answers and came up with none, what about the parents who don't know where to look or what questions to ask?

Nine years ago, I had no idea that one day I would be starting a soap manufacturing business, appearing in the media, or writing a book. That was not what I had in mind during the nine months of my pregnancy. Before David was born, I saw myself as the mom who would be going to play dates, not to board meetings. I was the mom who would be baking cookies and cakes, not overseeing the ingredients, labeling, and packaging of a product line. I have always had a love for people and for children and knew I was happy and comfortable doing the "touchy feely" thing with friends and family. I never thought I'd be sharing on radio and television talk shows my personal battles and private frustrations in my struggle to heal my son. I now believe that my life's calling is to be the mom among the big companies that dominate the multi-billion-dollar chemical industry and to be the small voice that haunts the manufacturers of chemical-laden products in their corporate buildings.

*Why David Hated Tuesdays* is an opportunity for me to pass along what I have learned about chemicals, hidden toxins, and alternative products and to help you reorganize your home to be as human- and earth-friendly as possible. I certainly do not have all the answers, and I am not an expert on *your* situation, but this book—my journey—may help you find your own answers, your personal strength, your "yes, I can do this!" voice.

All that you will read here I learned through the mistakes, challenges, obstacles, and tears of the past 10 years. As a result of my experiences, I feel a strong need to "talk to you" about the choices that we make in our homes and in our lives that can greatly impact us and our loved ones. That sounds like pretty "big stuff," but experience is a great educator.

I invite you to join me as, together, we look at your home and make some changes and choices from a new perspective, all in the name of creating a home that truly is "home sweet home."

# How to Use This Book

**W**HY DAVID HATED TUESDAYS is a guide to help you take steps to make your home as free of chemicals as you choose it to be. I repeat—as you choose it to be. In my case, because of my son's multiple chemical sensitivities, there were some areas where I had no choice. For example, I had to get rid of the carpeting in my house, and I could no longer wear synthetic fabrics or clothes that required dry cleaning or use detergent.

Only you can make the choices that work best for you and your family. Only you know how much or how little you need or want to change your home. Only you know what your boundaries and limits are in making change.

I promise you that this book will make you look at your home and your life differently. It takes you on my journey, so you can see through my eyes how I began to understand the unconscious choices I was making in my life. You will see the autopilot decisions I made that resulted in me bringing unsafe products and toxins into my home. You will see how I began to make the link between these decisions and my son's illness. Most of the changes I made to our home and lifestyle occurred during David's first five years; but even today I ask myself what I can do better. I'll never be "done" making David's environment as healthy as I can. However, I've learned not to expect perfection; all we can do is our best.

This book, in which we "get back to basics," provides you with the tools for taking a journey to a safer home and a healthier, human-friendly environment. These tools include the following:

- instructions on how to keep a journal to help you in the process of discovery and change
- questions to ask yourself about your home
- questions to ask when purchasing furnishings and other household items
- tips for finding out what is in your products
- resources and references for valuable information if you choose to dig deeper into a topic

The appendix lists the companies, authors, products, and more cited throughout this book that can help you maintain a healthy and organized home.

## The Journal

It was by keeping a journal that I discovered what was making David ill. I've filled countless journals since learning the value of this tool. Our lives are not stationary, and keeping a journal can help us focus our thoughts and figure out how to deal with the changes that come into our lives. In writing a journal as this book suggests, you'll literally track your life, your thoughts, what happens day to day, how you feel, when you are up and when you are down. It is a written document that validates you. My journal was where I saw that the doctors were wrong, where I could track when David was okay and when he got worse. This was where I could see the anxious moments in my life. It is there right in front of you. You can't fix a problem if you don't know what the problem is. The journal can help you discover your challenges. Your choice, at that point, becomes how and if you want to make a change. It all starts with the journal.

When you record what actually occurs in a room, you may be amazed by what you learn. I've gone into hundreds of homes, at people's request, to help them find out what was wrong. When I suggest that we look at how they organize their home as we search for toxins, the first thing they say—sometimes with indignation—is that they are already organized and that their home is free of chemicals. They think, as I did, that if they make it through the day, everything is fine. However, when we begin to define and organize room by room, we find old products, knickknacks that collect dust, toxic product residue on surfaces, and much more that is harmful to the family's health and slows them down. People are always stunned. Your observations in your journal may stun you, too, into saying, "Is that what is really happening in this room?" or "Did I just see that?" Your goal for each room cannot help but become crystal clear! So yes, I am going to strongly suggest that for a productive makeover of the rooms in your home, you're going to have to do some homework. Only then will you truly be in control and aware of how toxins creep into our lives.

The way the journal process works is that in each room of your house, you ask a series of questions and record your answers in your journal. Begin writing the journal using whatever method is comfortable for you. Would you rather jot things down that go on in the house hour by hour and day by day, or would you prefer to focus on the happenings in one room at a time? Or you can just write in your journal when a thought pops into your head. Even this style of documenting your life will begin to show you some rights and wrongs. Just begin writing. There is no right or wrong way.

I've devoted a chapter to each room of the house and provided you with journal questions specific to that room. Answering these questions will help you determine what changes might be appropriate or necessary for you and your family to create a healthier environment. Do not limit your questions to those I have asked. Remember, this is your home, and you have your own needs, styles, likes, and dislikes. To make this healthy makeover work, each room has to serve the users' needs. For example, my place of relaxation from the stress of the day is my bathroom, so in addition to ridding this room of toxins, I needed to make sure that it was "me," which means no children's toys, no partner's bathrobe, no clutter.

If a journal is just way too much for you and the idea of me asking you to keep a journal will make you put the book down right here, let's take it down one notch. Make a list. List every room in your home, and next to each room write the purpose that you would like that room to fill. Perhaps your desire for the living room is a place to quietly watch television and have the kids play nearby. Your bedroom is to be a place where you and your partner can connect at the end of the day. This way as you move through the book, you at least have something in front of you, in black and white, that shows your customized choices for your home, what functions well in a given room, and what toxic products and furnishings you need to remove.

If that is still too much for you, get a sticky pad and attach a note to each door or entrance to every room in your home. As you go about your day, jot down on the note what is going on in that room. If you feel you already know what is going on in each of your rooms, write the purpose of each room on the sticky note, attach the note to the door or entrance, and observe for a day how accurate you are. Defining the purpose for each room helps you see how effective your environment is in helping you move through life. If the day of observation reveals that your rooms are not serving the purpose you thought they were, remember, becoming aware is half the battle.

Once you have information and a true picture of a room's current use, you have the facts to make decisions for you and your family. You know what happens, when it happens, and how it happens in that room. You have gained insight into how you feel in each room. Without a journal or some documentation, trying to remember all the details of a day, let alone a week, is impossible. It can be even harder to pinpoint if problems such as chronic sneezing or puffy red eyes occur in the morning, noon, or night or in a specific area of the house. A journal is a great detective's tool!

If there are others in your household, don't take on this project of redefining, reorganizing, and cleaning all by yourself. Invite them onto your team! I have discovered, in both my business and my personal life, that bringing others into the process is a wonderful way for them to change their ways of doing things and accept the changes around them.

If you are interested in the team approach to the journal, it is critical that "your team" know and understand the importance of having a home that is a healthy environment, as free of harmful toxins as possible. In other words, "What's in it for them?" If you can explain to them how this project can help them as well as you, then they are more apt to get involved. You'll also be teaching them some wonderful life skills—teamwork, cooperation, compromise, and, just perhaps, "a job well done." Since they will have a deciding vote, or at least some input, it keeps complaints about all the changes to a minimum. (I said minimum; don't think all the whining will go away.)

And finally, if you are a control freak (and I say that with affection) and if you are used to doing it all, perhaps now is a good time to learn how to ask for help. You'll be amazed at how uplifting it is to lighten your load.

## "Good, Better, Best" Boxes

In the process of trying to make my whole house safe, sometimes I was beside myself, wailing, "How am I going to do this!" At some point you will probably become overwhelmed too. For this reason I present Good, Better, Best boxes throughout the book. These boxes offer choices—specific actions—that you can take to create a safer environment. You can make changes immediately or make changes in stages, beginning with the simplest and moving to the more complicated or costly. Sometimes the choices in the Good, Better, Best boxes are cumulative; you can do all three steps, if you desire, with Best being the most complete action. In other cases, the Good, Better, Best actions are either-or choices.

For example, if you have determined that the dining room is only used for special occasions and is generally closed off from day-to-day living, then perhaps it can be listed as "less priority" or "limited changes," or maybe "it's just right" the way it is!

Even if you choose to do nothing but read the book, you'll come away from it knowing what the primary chemicals are in your home and where they are hidden—and trust me, you will look at bedding, furnishings, and household products with a much more critical eye.

## Good, Better, Best: **Keeping the Journal**

**Good:** You and your family put up sticky notes in each room and record the purpose, issues, and concerns of each room as things come to mind.

**Better:** You write the journal by asking the questions and observing how each room is used over a period of time.

**Best:** Everybody who uses a room keeps his or her own journal, and then all ideas are brought together for a general consensus on how the makeover of all the rooms in the house should take place.

# *"Better Choice Mom Recommends" Information*

You'll also see information labeled "Better Choice Mom Recommends." This is my chance to bring to your attention practical products that work, as well as Web sites, books, and reports that you may find of use. Why the name "Better Choice Mom"? I chose it because it fits my passion so well: helping other mothers wade through the information (and misinformation) out there and empowering them to choose what's best for their family.

Now that you are ready to take on "the fight," begin by recognizing that the toxic issues in your home will not be resolved in a day, a week, or even a month. Changes may be small and progress slow, but if you take this opportunity to make changes or become more aware of the issues described in the book, I guarantee that the rewards will be great, and you will feel good knowing that you've created a healthier environment for your loved ones. I promise you that!

# Foreword

I HAVE BEEN A PEDIATRICIAN for over 40 years, practicing in Buffalo, New York, until I moved to Scottsdale, Arizona. Here, I have continued to study, research, and write about the chemicals and pollutants harming our environment and thus harming ourselves, our children, and a generation of children to come.

Through my work, I have met many a parent with children suffering from toxins and allergies to food, mold, and dust. One of those parents I had the good fortune to meet was Amilya Antonetti. It was apparent when we met that Amilya was in no way going to stand by patiently and wait for what *might be* answers. If no one could help, then she would do it herself. She did not wait; and she did find answers.

What makes Amilya a truly inspirational person is that she has taken her passion and commitment to her son and channeled it into a commitment to help others. I admire her as an entrepreneur, a trailblazer in the billion-dollar soap industry, and a mother whose passion to do for others has never wavered.

This book, written for anyone who wants to make their home a healthier environment for themselves and their loved ones, has been written with her unbridled enthusiasm and her desire to help others so that not one parent has to endure seeing the pain and suffering she saw in her infant son's eyes.

Amilya is a gift, as is this book she offers you.

—*Doris Rapp, M.D.*

# CHAPTER 1

# Amilya and David's Story

## A Journey to Health

You gain strength, courage, and confidence by every experience in which you really stop to look fear in the face. You are able to say to yourself, "I have lived through this horror. I can take the next thing that comes along." You must do the thing you think you cannot do.

—Eleanor Roosevelt

THE DAY I BROUGHT MY newborn son home from the hospital was perfect. The blue sky matched the color of my infant son's eyes. A warm breeze ruffled David's fine, dark hair and carried his sweet scent out into the world. I felt even more complete than I had imagined I would after months of caring for myself and my baby as he grew inside me and I joyfully anticipated his homecoming.

But my joy was muted by David's incessant crying, which filled our days and nights. His screams were chilling, an indication of real pain and suffering. He began to experience shortness of breath and a dry, hacking cough, which often kept both of us up at night. He developed chronic skin problems, including raised, scablike rashes that appeared on different parts of his body. Sometimes when I removed his diaper or t-shirt, his skin would peel off in sheets. He had a swollen, red ring around his bottom that made diapering a nightmare: Though I was as gentle as possible, he'd bleed as I wiped his little tushie, and he'd cry with pain the entire time. Other symptoms, which developed over the beginning months of his life, included itchy skin, gasping for breath, glassy eyes, dripping nose, and endless crying.

I felt helpless. What was wrong with my baby? What was I doing wrong that I could not help him and stop his crying?

Unable to answer these questions, my world was loud—with my own restless thoughts and the continuous advice of family and friends, offered out of kindness and concern—yet silent at the same time because nothing worked for David.

My bursting heart was now a broken heart. The euphoria of David's arrival was replaced with a tidal wave of fear. All I knew was that my son, the most precious gift I had ever received, was in agony, and nothing I did seemed to ease his suffering.

After a few days of David's nonstop crying, I took him to his pediatrician instead of waiting for his two-week checkup as I had been instructed to do. I looked to the doctor, whom I viewed as the expert, to tell me what was wrong with David and why I wasn't being a good mother; why my baby cried all the time; and why he wasn't a normal, healthy pink color like other babies. (He was a grayish color, and his skin was scaly, almost lizardlike.)

Over the next month, we took numerous trips to the pediatrician to relieve David's shortness of breath and skin issues. The quest to discover the source of his skin sensitivities led to consultations with specialists and more specialists, who took X rays, drew blood, and ran urine tests; allergists gave David the "poke test." In one month, David had seen more doctors and undergone more tests than I had in my entire life. They found nothing, and I still had no answers for what was the matter with my baby.

At first, the pediatrician told me, "Some babies have a tough time adjusting in the beginning." When the first month had passed and David was still crying, he said, "It's colic. It will last four to six months." After six months of David's screaming, I heard, "First-time moms tend to overreact. Relax and he will get better with time," and the best one of all, "This is hurting you more than it is hurting him."

Doctors, nurses, specialists—everyone I consulted—talked over me, around me, and to anyone else but me as I watched my baby gasping for air. Each time he had a severe attack, I ended up taking him to the emergency room. The doctors would hook him up to a respirator or give him inhalers, all to help him "get through this." During regular office visits, trips to the emergency room, appointments with dermatologists and allergists, tests done at the lab, and follow-up appointments with the specialists, I seemed to be the only one saying, "I don't want to just get him through this. I want his suffering to end."

"Deal with it" was not an option for me. "Live with it" was unlivable.

The worst piece of advice of all, the one that shook me to the core, came from a pediatric specialist who advised, "Let him go. You are young and can have more children."

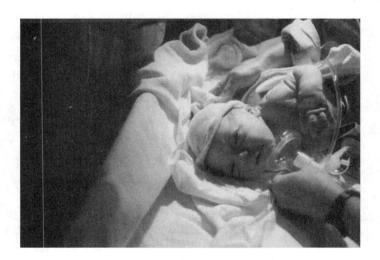

Was this to be my child's life? At six weeks old, David had to be given oxygen just to help him breathe.

I sat in his office, stunned by these words. I thought, "This is an expert?" "How much did I just pay to hear that I should let my son die?" No matter how many degrees he had, no one was going to convince me not to fight for my son's life.

It was at that point that I said "stop." I decided that having doctors put my son on a respirator until he was "well," only to have David return for treatment with the exact same symptoms a week later, was not good enough. This was not an answer. In my mind, there had to be a *reason* for his illnesses, not just temporary relief.

Since it appeared that the specialists could not find an answer, nor were they willing to take the time to search for what was wrong with my son, it was up to me. I decided then and there that I was going to do everything I could to find the answers that the medical community could not. I decided it was better to fight to the end and lose than never to fight at all. Trust me, there is nothing like the determination, power, and drive of an angry, frustrated mother!

## Taking Control

I began to take responsibility for being a bystander when it came to my son's health and hoping that the experts might know what was best for my son. I had allowed them to make all the decisions. What was I thinking? I was his mother. I had to do something! Though the doctors had the desire, unfortunately what was afflicting David wasn't "run-of-the-mill," and training in the area of what I now know as environmental illness/multiple chemical sensitivity wasn't taught in medical school. Many were as baffled as I was! I committed myself to finding a way to help David. I took back control and decisionmaking from family and friends and from the doctors, nurses, specialists, and other experts to whom I had given it.

If there was any way I could prevent it, I was not going to have my son going through life in pain, dependent on inhalers, being labeled as sickly or not normal. If I could help it, there would be no more heart-stopping trips to hospital emergency rooms. I embraced the power that comes from desperation and turned my deep pain and anger into the energy to fight back.

When I stopped looking outward for the answers and began making my own choices, things began to change for David and for me. I no longer accepted pat answers and more medications. I "pushed back" at the doctors, asking why. For instance, when I read the drug information on cortisone, which had been prescribed, and learned it should be taken for just 10 days, I asked the doctor why David had been on it for 10 weeks. I asked if there were alternatives to prescription drugs. I realized that when it came to David's illnesses, they just didn't have answers. Though I continued to take David to doctors and keep him on the medicines they prescribed, I began to understand that although parts of David were challenged (lungs and skin), the rest of him was strong. I could help his body and mind by giving them what they needed in the way of food, water, light, and rest while I researched and learned how to support the areas of him that were weak.

I became a mother on a quest. I subscribed to every health and medical magazine I could find. I read physicians' reference books. I uncovered every theory about shortness of breath and aggravated skin problems. I gained insight and received a great deal of comfort and inspiration by talking with other parents in hospitals and doctors' waiting rooms. On their advice and through my reading, I opened myself to the idea of alternative treatments.

A visit to a homeopathic doctor made me reexamine how I had been dealing with David's afflictions, both by my actions (trips to the experts) and by my emotional and mental response. The conventional doctors had shown me, by their lack of a diagnosis, that it was not going to be simple to find out what was wrong with David. The homeopathic doctor emphasized that what I was looking for was "a needle in a haystack," with the needle being potentially fatal for David.

It also became quite clear that even though David was not physically in my womb, my connection to him was just as strong as if he were still attached by the umbilical cord. I understood then that if I allowed myself to fuss, "freak out," or show anxiety, David would feel it too.

Though I still didn't have an answer as to what was making my son ill, these realizations were the first steps in taking charge. They started me doing something productive for him and not just driving him to doctor's appointments and to labs for more tests. To chronicle the details of David's life and how I was feeling and responding to his illness, I began keeping a journal. Since I was a walking zombie much of the time because of sleep deprivation and the emotional and psychological trauma of David's illness, I couldn't recall what I had had for breakfast, let alone remember the details from one day to the next. The journal was a must if I was really going to find out what was happening in our lives. To find the needle in the haystack, I needed to know what parts of the haystack I had searched through already. The journal became my first ally and tool in a fight against my unknown enemy.

## A Journal of Discovery

I wrote down what David ate, what he wore, when he slept, when he was happy, when he was in pain, and just important, how I was handling his crisis. A pattern emerged in the journal: David hated Tuesdays. He always ended up sick on that day.

What happened in our house on Tuesday? Was it the food? I always ate meat loaf on Tuesdays, so was it something in the meat loaf passed to David through my breast milk? After a month of journaling, trying to unravel the problem with Tuesdays, the revelation came to me.

Along with making meat loaf on Tuesdays, I also pulled out the tile cleaner, the floor cleaner, the counter cleaner, the window cleaner, the toilet bowl tablets, and the carpet freshener. A light went on in my head. Could the itchy skin, swollen and red-ringed bottom, gasps for breath, glassy eyes, dripping nose, dry coughs, and endless crying be connected to this array of ultrastrong household cleaners that I spread around my house every Tuesday?

I did not clean that morning but instead wrote down all the ingredients listed on the label of each product I used to clean. The words were foreign to me. What were propylene, glycol, lauryl polyglucose, and methychlorosothizolione, and what were they doing in my liquid soap? My next big discovery was that some products didn't even list ingredients. Did this mean that as a "good" consumer I had blindly trusted that these products were safe?

Baby in arms, I headed to the library and pulled books on cleaning and chemicals from the shelves. In one book I found a description of something called "environmental illness," which talked about some of the chemicals on my list and the destructive things they do to the body, many of which matched David's symptoms. Another book I found, *Is This Your Child? Discovering and Treating Unrecognized Allergies in Children and Adults,* by Doris J. Rapp, M.D., also described David's condition and showed pictures of babies and children who looked just like my son: dark circles under the eyes, red ears, a glassy-eyed expression, and skin rashes. All these conditions were attributed to chemicals.

In a panic at what I saw and what I began to learn from the books about harmful chemicals in cleaning products, I rushed home and threw out everything under my kitchen sink, in my laundry room, and in my bathroom. Then I opened the windows, sat down, and cried tears of relief. Finally, perhaps I had found an answer. But could this really be? Could things so common to everyone's households be causing my son's many health issues?

Miraculously, David did not get sick that day or any day in the next week. The sink was loaded with dirty dishes, and the floor was piled with dirty laundry, but my friends and family were celebrating because my baby son was sleeping through the night for the first time in his life. The house was so quiet you could almost hear the tears rolling down my face.

## Becoming a Better Choice Mom

This first revelation that chemicals were the culprit only spurred me to find out more. It was as if a fire had been lit in me. Even as I learned more about the hazards of chemicals, where they hide in our homes, and the damage they can cause, I kept thinking, How can this be?

Even though somewhat of a "clean freak," I let the cleaning go during this time. Of course I knew that the house was going to have to be cleaned eventually, but with what? I searched for alternative cleaning products that were not toxic, that did not have foreign-sounding ingredients, and that did not list harmful physical side effects. What I found were products sold mainly at health food stores (meaning an additional stop on shopping day). They were more expensive than what I could purchase at the grocery store, and when I tried them out, I found that they did not clean very well. Obviously, my crusade to give David a happier, healthier life had many more steps before completion.

I discovered that the "soaps" we use today are made from synthetics created in a lab. So I reached back in time to our grandmothers and great-grandmothers and collected recipes from the days when people, not companies, made cleaning products. I began to brew different concoctions in my kitchen sink. The result was a bar of soap that did not aggravate David's skin condition. Another victory!

Now what to do about the dishes he ate off and the sheets he slept on? Back to the drawing board. I tried using a cheese grater to make the bar of soap into powder. It took several attempts to get the soap fine enough to dissolve in water. Once I achieved that, I combined the soap flakes with vinegar and citrus zest from lemons and oranges to make liquid soap. I also experimented with essential oils and different bases (oil, water), all in the name of making a healthy home for my son.

Slowly, I began to narrow down what worked well in my home and what worked for David. The more information I gathered, the more I could then tweak the original soap flakes recipe so that I could use it all over the house on different surfaces and in different ways.

When friends, neighbors, and family came to visit, I would show them my "soap brewery." I initially made a joke out of it, using it as an excuse for the condition of my kitchen, with pots, molds, graters, herbs, and citrus fruit as my main staples in lieu of bread, coffee, and milk.

When they saw how well David was doing (no peeling skin or rash, red eyes, or swollen glands), they said it was a miracle. I responded that it was no miracle; it was the soap and the back-to-basics approach I was now taking to clean my house. Naturally, wanting them to share in my happiness and discovery, I invited them to try it and see what it did for them.

Though I was very pleased with my success, I still had doubts about whether this was really the answer to David's health problems. I needed to know if I was the only mother out there who had a child who was not going to be able to do sleepovers, eat cafeteria food, or go on scouting trips. I needed answers, and I needed support. I was Ms. Suburbia, and I liked my life. I did not want to turn David or myself into "granola crunchers" and wheat grass drinkers. I knew if I had found one answer—chemicals in the cleaning products—there had to be more answers. What I had learned only drove me to continue my quest.

I began by inviting anyone and everyone—other mothers, people I met in doctors' waiting rooms, people from the grocery store and pharmacy—over to my house to try the products I was making in my home.

I then took it one step further by placing an advertisement—"Calling All Moms"—in the *Penny Saver,* a free newspaper in my area. It read, "Bring your children. Meet other moms. Discuss health issues of your child." This was my way of reaching out to real moms about what was going on with our children. A local hotel donated the room, and a caterer donated the food. Over 200 parents responded to the ad and showed up for the three-hour meeting. What a shock! The big response showed me that David was not the only child who was suffering and that I was not alone.

Today I recognize that what I was doing was starting a support group for mothers of sick children, some of whom had multiple chemical sensitivities. For me, it was just a get-together. When we met, sometimes at the park or many times over the kitchen sink, grating soap while our children played in the backyard, we shared stories of how we used socks and nylons over our children's hands to stop their relentless scratching and how the pain of their sores and skin penetrated into our very souls. We all were frustrated with the steroid creams and hydrocortisone ointments that did nothing about the cause of our children's agony but only masked the problem. The horror stories we shared, the tears we shed, and the inspiration we gave one another were exactly what I needed. But again, I knew there was more work to be done if any of us were going to be the June Cleavers we had envisioned being.

My moms' network grew as word of my soap spread to other mothers who had children with skin sensitivities. All were amazed that I was just "whipping this up" in my kitchen sink. I too was amazed, but because of their encouragement and my ongoing self-education in the world of chemicals (or perhaps out of sheer naïveté), I thought I could do better than make soap in my sink.

## A Company with a Cause

In November 1995, when David was around two years old, I started Soapworks, a company that makes and distributes nontoxic natural

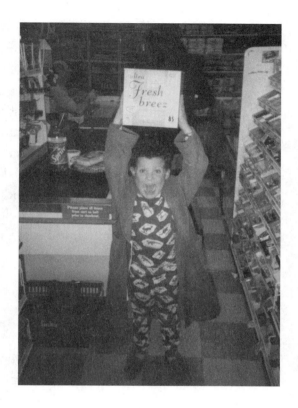

David, age five, celebrates seeing "his mommy's product" at the store. (He'd just come from the hospital, where he'd been receiving treatment for an asthma attack triggered by inhaling toxins at school.)

soap made from a vegetable base and using the natural cleaning power of oxygen and citrus. As much as I wanted to offer a great product, it was also important to me to be a voice for mothers. I wanted to inform other mothers of the dangers of believing that what is on the grocery store shelf is safe to use. I had learned the hard way that what was most convenient and on sale might not be the best choice for my family. It was my hope that by launching Soapworks and through the example of my own personal struggle, I could help other families and especially other children like David.

In the process of setting up this business, I made all kinds of discoveries that convinced me to continue my research and study of toxins in the home. I thought, "Sure, Soapworks provides wonderful alternatives to mainstream cleaning products, but what about all the other chemicals and toxins that are in our homes? Are people really aware of their hazards and the harm they can cause?" I highly doubted it since I had been amazed and shocked at the information I had discovered that first day in the library. I continued to be wide-eyed with horror by what I discovered on a daily basis.

At that point, I reexamined my commitment to David, which was to make his life better. On one level, I had done that: His health was better. But was that all there was to the commitment to my son? He still had to go out and participate in a world that could be very harmful to him. It was clear that I could not keep the knowledge about our chemical-saturated world to myself.

## Spreading the Word

If in a parenting class, breast-feeding class, or safety tips program for parents I had been informed about chemicals or even given a "heads-up" about the possible dangers, maybe I would have been more prepared and would have started to explore my options much sooner. With the knowledge I had gained, I was now in a position to provide the heads-up. If in doing so I could spare one family from the anguish that my family had suffered watching David struggle for two years, then I had to do something beyond producing hypoallergenic, nontoxic cleaning products. Soapworks would be my voice to help me raise the flag, ring the bell, and sound the alarm about toxins and chemicals. My quest now was to go beyond Soapworks production and create a mom-to-mom network to take the place of the extended families that existed generations ago.

As my group of moms grew and my voice traveled through their voices, I was invited to do a radio interview to tell my story. With a nervous belly and sweaty palms, I took to the airways to speak to other moms to let them know that they were not alone, they were not crazy, and there were answers to help them. I shared the information I had learned with hundreds of listeners and gave concrete answers to real questions such as what else is out there for toothpaste and what to use for wipes, bedding, clothing, makeup, and more. I referred callers to companies like mine that were trying to make a difference. Not only did I give information, but my newfound family shared with me things they had learned and companies they had come across. My extended family was growing and on the move!

From my local radio appearances, word slowly spread, and I was invited to do more and more radio talk shows telling David's and my story as well as answering listeners' questions. With each step, I was overwhelmed at the response—and the need. I was embraced by so many wonderful moms who helped cheer me forward. Their "you go, girl" support told me that I had made the right decision in going forth with Soapworks as well as in offering a shoulder to cry on, via mass media, for other parents frustrated with mainstream medical practices and with commercial products.

When I was asked to make my first television appearance on a local morning talk show, the thought made me nervous to the point of being sick, but I knew that this was a wonderful opportunity to reach out to many more moms.

Over the past eight years, the exposure on such television shows as *Extra, Sally Jesse Raphael, CBS This Morning,* and, most recently, *Oprah* has been wonderful. I've also spread the word through magazine stories in *Time, People,* and *Working Mother.* Some shows want to talk about David and the drama of the illness. Others want answers about what deodorant to use or if coloring your hair will cause cancer. Producers and editors began calling me "The Better Choice Mom" because on each show, I offered viewers and listeners practical choices. The name stuck.

Now more than ever I believe that everyone has the life he or she was meant to live. Did I think I was going to be a soap manufacturer? No. Did I think I would be the voice among many moms? No. And to tell you the truth, I still cannot believe I am "Amilya the soap maker" and now "The Better Choice Mom"—when all I wanted to be was a mom. Being a soap manufacturer, however, gave me the tools—and the media gave me the vehicle—to share what I have learned about toxins, chemicals, and what lurks in our homes. For this opportunity, I will be forever grateful, and with all the joys this new journey has brought me, I never start a single day without feeling and remembering where this all began—with the birth of my precious son, David.

The fact that I might have a son with physical challenges never entered my mind when I was pregnant. This journey was not my choice. But what it did was give me a calling, one that I never would have found by attending college or in any career in the corporate world. I've learned that ignorance is *not* bliss.

Being able to ride your own wave, to make choices that are absolutely suited to you and your family, is empowering. Through this book, I pass on to you the opportunity to embrace the power of making positive choices for your family. And, one home at a time, we can make the world a safer place for our children.

# CHAPTER 2

# Home Sweet Home— or Is It?

## Issues That Affect the Entire House

I am only one, but still I am one. I cannot do everything, but still I can do something; and because I cannot do everything, I will not refuse to do something that I can do.
　　—Edmund Everett Hale

WHEN THE SWITCH FINALLY WENT ON and I realized that common household products were contributing to the slow poisoning of my child, I immediately wanted to tackle everything. I felt that turning my home upside down, throwing everything away, and starting from scratch was the only answer. My fear for my son's life was matched only by my frustration and anger at discovering the truth about my "happy home." I was shocked when I finally began to understand that virtually everything in my home, from cleansers to carpets, even resealable plastic containers and bags, was potentially dangerous to my family and me.

Since I didn't know that my home could be a "danger zone," I did not alter the way I had lived as a single person when I got married or when I became pregnant. My rationale for continuing my lifestyle was that I had made it this far in life drinking colas, eating fast food, and taking Martha Stewart's decorating advice (yikes—glue guns!). I wore whatever was in style regardless of the fabric or cleaning requirements without suffering any side effects, so what was the problem?

I had no idea that these everyday choices had any negative consequences except the inconvenience of having to go to the dry cleaners or maybe a few unwanted pounds from one too many Big Macs. Why would I even look at labels or ingredients or be concerned about what was being sprayed in my yard? I was young and healthy, and I didn't think getting married or having a baby meant I needed to change anything. Of course, I did the mommy-to-be things like eating the right foods, taking additional vitamins, and attending parenting classes. I really didn't think there was much else I needed to do to make sure I delivered a healthy baby and made a healthy, happy home for him.

If I had been the one suffering, I probably would have popped a pill, taken another sick day, and attributed it to "age catching up with me." But it was my son who lay helpless, and now the "deal with it" mentality that I had previously used for me to plow through a day despite feeling lousy and the "live with it" answers that I got from my doctors regarding my son were no longer acceptable.

I had to acknowledge that the toxins I'd brought into my home were what had set off David's medical problems. I also had to come to the realization that David would have had a happier, healthier beginning in life if I had just been more aware of these "toxic creeps" and known of the available alternatives before he came home from the hospital.

Before I was able to begin making better choices for my family, I needed to understand the big picture, to examine the tangibles (desks, carpeting, shower curtains, and all) and the intangibles (the air and the environment) that were affecting David's life. Carefully considering everything in our surroundings helped me understand that wall-to-wall carpeting, poor ventilation, the water system, and even the structure of my home were potentially all culprits. Though I wanted to, I knew I couldn't rebuild my house from the ground up. What I *could* do was change the kind of products we used, from cleansers to shampoo and toothpaste. With these small changes, I began to take back the power I had given away. I took the first steps to a healthy lifestyle.

## The Big Picture

Did you know that we are saturated in chemicals? We really are, and they can affect us each and every day.

There are simple changes you can make—today—in each room of your home that will make a difference to your health. This chapter discusses the main factors that can affect you and your family.

**Factors in the House That Affect Health**

- air quality
- lighting
- wall coverings
- carpeting
- dust control
- vacuum cleaners
- electromagnetic fields

## Air Quality

Before I began researching the subject, "air quality" in my home meant to me the smell of dinner cooking on the stove or brownies baking in the oven; "air pollution" meant something that happened outdoors in big cities. I knew about smog, car exhaust, and factory smoke, but I never thought twice about what that nastiness had to do with what I was breathing in my home.

In trying to discover all the things that might be affecting David, I read about legal battles waged by employees, schoolteachers, and parents of children who got sick when they returned to a building or school after remodeling, construction, or summer break. I now know that the use of toxic paints, sealants, and synthetics, in addition to poor ventilation, contributed to what is called "sick building syndrome." According to the Environmental Protection Agency (EPA), the concentrations of many pollutants are higher in indoor air than in outdoor air. Why is this? How did our buildings become sick?

Back in the "good old days," the construction of houses was a lot simpler than it is today. Fewer building materials were used in the construction of a house. Concrete, brick, asphalt, and real wood were pretty much it. Indoor furnishings were simpler too, with more natural products used, such as cotton, linen, and wool. Our schools had hardwood floors, wooden desks, and simple materials like paper, cardboard, and basic glue instead of plastic folders, binders, markers, and the adhesives in book binding. Buildings from that era also had lots of windows that could be opened as opposed to the permanently shut windows we often see in schools and buildings today. How many times do you stay in hotels and you can't open the window?

Windows in all buildings used to be regularly opened to let fresh air circulate! I cannot remember a single day that my grandma did not open up the whole house to let in the fresh air, even when we were yelling to her that it was snowing outside. As crazy as we thought she was, she was right. Fresh air makes a huge difference in our well-being.

So what happened to our homes, schools, and buildings? The problem began with the energy crunch of the 1970s, when people sealed their homes to conserve energy. As a result, people began recirculating the existing indoor air to control the temperature better and to save money. Hotels, schools, office and community buildings,

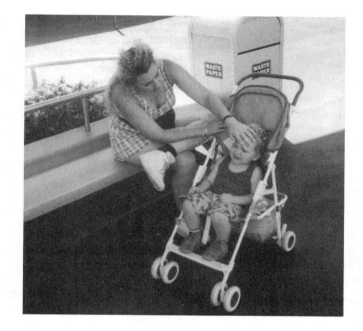

No matter how fussy David was, I always made sure we went out for a walk, no matter the weather or how he or I felt.

and other buildings quickly followed suit. The consequence was a lessening in air exchange with the fresh outside air, so more toxins and germs were trapped inside. An example of this occurs on airplanes, where the same air, including the germs, is recirculated for the entire flight. That means you're breathing the germs of the gentleman nearby who just sneezed *and* the woman in the back of the plane who is having a coughing fit. No wonder many of us become sick after we travel by air.

In an airplane, it is necessary to recirculate air; in our homes, it is just cheaper. We sacrifice air quality in our homes for lower electric bills. My question is this: If the resulting concentration of toxins and germs is a direct cause of us being sicker, are we really saving money, or are we just paying for bad air? Some trade-off!

Since the lungs are usually the first organs to be affected and since most of us do not suffer immediate symptoms, you may not make the connection that illnesses—colds, flu, allergies, bronchitis, headaches, fatigue, stress, and anxieties—may be the result of the poor air quality in your own home.

The dramatic increase in chemicals used in the manufacture of building materials, furnishings, fabrics, carpets, and household cleaning and personal care products has also had a large impact on indoor air. Our homes are now filled with synthetic materials and chemicals, in everything from the carpets our kids play on to the pajamas they sleep in. These synthetic materials have been treated with flame retardants, fungicides, pesticides, and biocides (a chemical agent, such as a pesticide, capable of destroying living organisms)—all of which we trap tightly in our homes, never thinking that they could be the source of the illnesses from which one or more of our family members suffer.

The more you become aware of all the sources of chemicals in your home, the more you can do to reduce the amount of toxins around you and improve the air quality for your whole family. Here is an equation to keep in mind:

**more airtight houses + less air exchange + more synthetics + more chemicals = toxic air and bad health**

What exactly is in our indoor air? Here's a partial list: dust mites; molds; pet dander; pollen; combustion by-products; tobacco smoke; chemical outgassing (toxins released into the air by synthetic products, also called off-gassing) from home improvements like carpeting, wallpaper, paint, shelving, and household products; bacteria and viruses; trace metals; and pesticides. And you thought you were safe!

## Air Filtration

There isn't much we can do about the poor quality of outdoor air, but there are plenty of options for improving the air inside your home. If you have centralized heat or an air-conditioning system, one of the simplest things you can do is this: Make sure there are good filters on the intake and output vents. Be aware that the filters that the manufacturer installed in the central heat/air unit are there to protect the unit. They're not there to protect your health. To make a difference in your health, you must upgrade the filters to capture such things as dust, pollen, and volatile organic compounds (VOCs) and other carcinogens. (A carcinogen is a chemical known or believed to cause cancer in humans.)

Although plain filters have been on the market for years, today there are higher-grade filters available. The most common types use activated carbon, mechanical filtration (HEPA, which stands for "high-efficiency particulate arresting"), electrostatic filtration, or negative-ion filtration. They range in price from $2 to $20 and can be found in most hardware and home improvement stores, whose employees will usually be happy to advise you on how to change the filter.

Regardless of the type of filter you choose, you must remember to replace them often. The filters will have a manufacturer recommendation on how often to change your filters, but you need to take into consideration your own lifestyle. Think about things such as how often you use the unit, how dusty the area is in which you live, and whether there are people with health challenges in your home. There is no more common mistake than forgetting about your filters. I suggest you put on your calendar when the manufacturer recommends you change the filter. It is that important.

Freestanding air filtering units for the individual rooms in your house can also be beneficial. It's important for this discussion to understand the difference between an air filter and an air purifier.

An *air filter* is simply a box with a motor that sucks air into it, filters the air, and blows it back out. When buying a unit, you have to know what each filter material is capable of taking out of the air. Many people buy a unit with fabric or foam filters, thinking that it will eliminate airborne chemicals such as formaldehyde. It will not. The air filtering device needs to have either activated charcoal filters to remove organic compounds, such as cooking odors, chemical odors, and smoke, or potassium permanganate filters for lighter gases, such as formaldehyde.

Once the filter is saturated, it will spit toxic material back into the air. This happens with most filters on any product. When the filter is full or blocked, the air has nowhere else to go. Filter replacement should be every 30 to 90 days, depending on where you live. If you are not someone who is likely to keep up with replacing filters, an air purifier might be a better option for you.

An *air purifier* uses ionization and ozone to clear particles and odors from the air. Air purifiers do not filter the air. The oxidizing action of ozone can kill bacteria and mold, eliminate odors, and break down chemicals. Ozone is now known to be one of the most powerful disinfectants and can kill microbial contaminants like *E. coli, Listeria, Salmonella, Giardia,* and *Cryptosporidium* more effectively than conventional disinfectants, such as chlorine. When ozone is added to the air, the particles in the air become heavy, causing the particles to fall from the air to the floor, where they can then be vacuumed up. Such units are designed to work in small areas. A common mistake is using a small unit to filter too large a room. Keep in mind that ozone is controversial because it can be irritating to the respiratory tract, though manufacturers of air purifiers that use ozone say the level is safe for everyday use. This is where keeping a journal and learning to become your own health detective is valuable.

In my home, I have a lot of open space and open rooms and was not able to find a single filtering unit capable of cleaning the air in the entire home. Most units can handle 800 to 1,500 square feet, and I needed more than one unit for my home. I resolved to get individual units for each room. Since this was going to be a costly endeavor and I couldn't do it all at once, I began by upgrading the filters in my heating and air-conditioning units and then putting an air purifier in David's room. In other rooms, I placed plants that take toxins out of the air. (See "Plants: Mother Earth's Natural Filters," page 24.) Over time, I got air purifiers for my bedroom and for each of the rooms in which we spent a lot of time.

As with replacing air filters for your central heating or air-conditioning unit, air filtering units range in quality as well as price. For optimal results, do not place the unit in front of or near windows or doors that are often open because the unit will then filter outside air entering your home as well as the inside air. A small, inexpensive air filtering unit can quickly become saturated with dust and particles, necessitating frequent changes of its filters.

When buying an air filter, shop around. Be sure to factor in the cost of the unit's filters and how often they need to be replaced. Many times people choose a less expensive unit, only to find out, much to their dismay, that the filters cost twice as much as those for competitive models.

Another air filtration option is to have a central air purification system professionally installed in your home. In these systems, the air is filtered by passing through several layers of filtration, including material that absorbs chemicals. Before investing in such a system, consult with an expert (in the yellow pages under heating air or ductwork) who can test your home air to determine what filtration needs are most important and what type of system is most suitable for your house. An assortment of systems at varying costs are available (see appendix for sources).

In considering air purifying units, you should know that some units work via ionization while others work via ozone. The most beneficial units employ both. There are a few points of caution regarding these units, however. Ozone can be irritating to some people. In addition, expecting an air purifier to do too big a job can also cause noxious chemicals to be released.

Further, many people who cannot afford to change all their furnishings think that they can simply buy an ozonator and "zap everything." This is an oversimplification. The unit can't solve all problems. If a carpet is so saturated with chemicals that it will outgas for 20 years, it needs to be removed. Use of an ozonator in such a case will only be a small bandage for a big problem.

If you run an air filter after people smoke, it may help clear the air of the smoke, but it may not get rid of the smell left in the furniture, curtains, and carpet. An air purifier can help in this regard, but it is only for occasional exposure. If someone smokes in the house every day, this is a bigger problem. Most air filters and purifiers have a tough time keep up with filtering out the amount of chemicals smoke releases.

I've never been a smoker, but both my parents and grandparents were. Although I have always hated smoke, I felt guilty about asking visitors to my home to go outside to smoke. I just tolerated it and then spent days airing out the house after they left. My dad didn't wait for me to tell him. A cigar smoker for years, he recognized that he would not be able to come over or hold David. That was incentive enough to quit. After I realized why David was sick, I got bolder. My rule became that all visiting smokers go outside. Then I didn't have to be concerned with them "messing up" the purifier with all the smoke when I needed the purifier to be used for the other toxins that I was trying to get out of my home. Today, nix on smoking even outside my house. It has taken me a while to get there, but I feel better and my son feels better.

### Plants: Mother Earth's Natural Filters

Not only do plants add a nice touch for the decor of your home, but they are quite useful in filtering the air. Plants, of course, take in carbon dioxide, which we exhale, and make oxygen; they also absorb other toxins. Doris Rapp, in *Is This Your Child's World?,* lists some common plants and their benefit:

| Plant Name | Toxins Removed |
| --- | --- |
| aloe vera | formaldehyde |
| elephant ear | formaldehyde |

| | |
|---|---|
| English ivy | benzene |
| ficus (weeping fig) | formaldehyde |
| golden pothos | carbon monoxide, benzene, formaldehyde |
| Janet Craig (corn plant) | benzene |
| peace lily | benzene trichloroethylene |
| spider plant | carbon monoxide |

## Air Ducts

Improperly installed, operated, or maintained heating and cooling systems can cause air quality problems. Air ducts are the tunnels that carry heated or cooled air from the main unit to each room. Dust, pollen, and other debris can accumulate in the ducts. If there is moisture, mold, and other microbes trapped in your ducts, they can grow easily, and you would never know it since most of us never even look into our ducts.

If you've never had the air ducts in your house cleaned, this is a definite "to do" in improving your air quality. A professional duct cleaning can reduce particulates in the house as well as increase the efficiency of your system. Since ductwork consists of a long tunnel, it is impossible to vacuum out the tunnel yourself. Professional companies that specialize in duct cleaning have the proper equipment to reach all the way through the duct to remove debris. After the initial cleaning, you'll need to check the ventilation system every year or do as I do and check with the changing of seasons. I feel so strongly about duct cleaning that it's the gift I always give to a new mother at a baby shower! No, it isn't very cute, but it is a gift of good health for the baby. A duct cleaning can cost anywhere from $100 to $250.

There are two clues that your ducts need a good cleaning. First, does your heater smell when you turn it on for the first time in autumn? Second, when you look at the air vents, the unit, and the intake vent, can you see a lot of dust in the first few feet? If so, you can feel pretty confident that the duct looks like that all the way through. Many companies offer a maintenance program. This is something to think about if the area you live in is very dusty or near a heavy manufacturing business or if you or other family members have severe health issues.

When I first had the ducts in my house cleaned, I was appalled at what the cleaners took out of the ducts. They showed me the dead mice, feces, and leftover toxic building materials in the ductwork. I didn't want to look at what we had been breathing, let alone think about how long we had been breathing it! After you get over the initial shock of what the professional cleaners find in the air ducts in your house, I don't think adding duct cleaning to your annual or seasonal "to do" list will be an issue.

A word about professional cleaning companies: Never allow people who work on the air ducts in your house to use biocides to kill organisms (insects, molds, dust mites, and so on) or to use a chemical sealant of any kind. These products can be disastrous to your health. Once sprayed, they can cause ill health effects, and, worse, the biocides are next to impossible to remove. Besides, believe it or not, they are unnecessary. With mold, for example, the solution is to find the cause, not to apply a quick fix. Unless the source of moisture is located and treated, it will be an ongoing problem. Sources of moisture can be leaks or improper installation. Cooling coils in air conditioning units can cause a buildup of condensation and moisture, so you must make sure the condensation pans are draining properly. If you have insulated air ducts and they have gotten wet or moldy, they cannot be cleaned and must be replaced.

## Good, Better, Best:  **Air Quality**

**Good:**  Be aware of how air quality affects your health. Circulate fresh air in your house as often as possible. Replace air filters on a regular basis as recommended for your units.

**Better:**  Upgrade the air filters, eliminate highly toxic materials in your home, and alternate between recirculating inside air and pulling in air from outside.

**Best:**  Have a central air purification unit installed in your house or place individual air purifiers in the main sleeping and living areas. Have exhaust fans installed in the kitchen and bathrooms and install a whole or partial house ventilation system (for example, HEPA).

For more information, you can contact the National Air Duct Cleaners Association (NADCA) or the Better Business Bureau.

# *Lighting*

Our bodies should be getting natural sunshine every day. I remember my grandmother sending us outside with the words, "Go out and blow the stink off!" Not getting enough sunlight, as in the winter months, can be a cause of a form of depression called seasonal affective disorder (SAD). (There are special lamps that emulate sunlight for treatment of SAD; see page 250 for information.)

Before the Industrial Revolution, people lived more in tune with nature. They got up at sunrise and started to wind down at sundown, just as we try to get our babies to do—awake during the day and sleeping (with any luck) through the night. The more we move away from the natural cycle of light by staying up late with artificial lighting, the greater the chances for health problems.

Many people can't or won't want to change their nighttime habits, but you can be aware of some alternatives for getting more natural light. For instance, if the weather in your area is nice, why not read the morning paper on the patio? If you go out to lunch from your office, walk rather than drive.

In considering the lighting in your home, one issue applies to all rooms: What type of lightbulb is best? Fluorescent lighting is increasingly being regarded as problematic. Though cost effective, fluorescent lighting fixtures produce an audible hum that has been connected to an increase in stress. They also have a fast flicker, which produces effects ranging from visual irritation to epileptic seizures. Studies have even linked skin rashes to fluorescent light. Artificial light overall has been associated with a decrease in calcium absorption, fatigue, decreased visual acuity, hyperactivity, restlessness, and even depression, as well as changes in heart rate, blood pressure, and the body's natural rhythms.

Fluorescent lights generate visible light by nonthermal mechanisms. Different kinds of light can be produced by adding phosphorus. Typically, the light produced by fluorescent light is a distorted spectrum of light that contains only a limited portion of the total spectrum. Cool-white light is deficient precisely in those areas of the spectrum where the sun's emission is the strongest. "The full-spectrum light, yielding the closest solar match in commercially available lighting, is perhaps state of the art in present day lighting technology," says Dr. Jacob Liberman in his book *Light Medicine of the Future*. Since most of us spend our waking hours indoors, it is important to be aware of how the lack of natural sunlight affects our health, productivity, and general well-being.

A strong relationship exists between light, our eyes, and our moods. The eyes alone use one-third as much oxygen as the heart and need 10 to 20 times as much vitamin C. Scientists have found that a significant relationship also exists between visual problems and mental illness. Their findings indicate that, while visual problems exist in only 9 percent of the general population, 66 percent of individuals suffering from depression, schizophrenia, or alcoholism have visual problems. Many other studies and reports conclude that light energy can influence the healing process and that the correct light source is critical to the normal functioning of the body.

As with many things, we are making progress with lighting. With the color balance of full-spectrum lighting and the three types of beneficial ultraviolet (UV) radiation that occur in the same proportions as in sunlight, man has come as close as possible to truly simulating natural sunlight.

The benefits of full-spectrum lighting include the following:

- reduction of glare, which in turn reduces eyestrain, headaches, fatigue, and irritability, thereby increasing productivity

- reduced levels of cortisol, the stress hormone

- no allergic skin reactions or dermatitis (Full-spectrum lighting can actually reduce such conditions.)

- slower aging process of the retina

- reduction in skin cancer

- general improvement in overall mood and feeling of well-being

By simply replacing fluorescent tubes with full-spectrum tubes, you can enhance your environment and your well-being. (Besides, fluorescent lights are so unflattering.) Hundreds of medical studies suggest the health benefits of UV light; however, the medical community still maintains that UV light is dangerous to our health. Natural full-spectrum lighting simulates the full color and UV spectrum of sunlight and reveals detail and color accurately. It is a beautiful, all-purpose white light—a tube that operates in existing fixtures for complete lighting of offices, stores, factories, schools, hospitals, banks, or wherever fluorescent light is used. Natural full-spectrum fluorescent lights have the proven capability to do the following:

- blend with natural light from windows and skylights

- reveal detail and colors accurately

- improve seeing

- improve the performance and productivity of people

- benefit pets and plants

Simulation of natural light means that light within a room can blend perfectly with the natural light from windows and skylights. The eye does not have to adapt to a new spectrum, color temperature, or color rendition when you go from outdoors to indoors. Also, interior colors are true.

Not all "full-spectrum" lightbulbs are true full spectrum. Lightbulbs are rated by lumen output (the amount of light they produce), CRI (color rendering index), and color temperature (degrees Kelvin). These ratings indicate the type of light the bulb is emitting. Natural light has a unique spectrum, which includes a balance of UV and visible color regions. This spectrum balance of UV and visible light is necessary for lamps to be called full spectrum. Therefore, if the spectrum from lightbulbs closely matches this balanced spectrum of natural noonday light, such bulbs can accurately and legitimately be described as full spectrum. Most so-called full-spectrum incandescent bulbs and neodymium are not true full spectrum and do not match high-quality full-spectrum lightbulbs.

Full-spectrum lightbulbs cost a few dollars more than regular lightbulbs but are worth it. Think of putting them in the areas of the house where family members read or study the most.

## Good, Better, Best:  **Lighting**

**Good:**    Be aware of how much time you spend outdoors each day. Try to get sunlight every day.

**Better:**    Change any fluorescent lightbulbs in your house to true full-spectrum bulbs.

**Best:**    Add natural light through skylights and glass blocks in your home.

## Better Choice Mom Recommends

The following Web sites are good sources of information on full-spectrum lightbulbs:

www.lightforhealth.com

www.sunformood.com

www.boltalightning.com

www.fullspectrumsolutions.com

www.truesun.com

# *Wall Coverings*

One of the activities that I find the most fun in decorating a house is deciding on wall coverings. Many of us get the "nesting" instinct when we are pregnant, and the first thing that comes to mind is wallpaper or paint, cute borders, and stick-on cartoon characters. Off we go to the store to find the right theme for the new baby's room. The problem is that while wallpaper, borders, painting, and stick-on pictures add color and personality to a room, they also, unfortunately, add toxins.

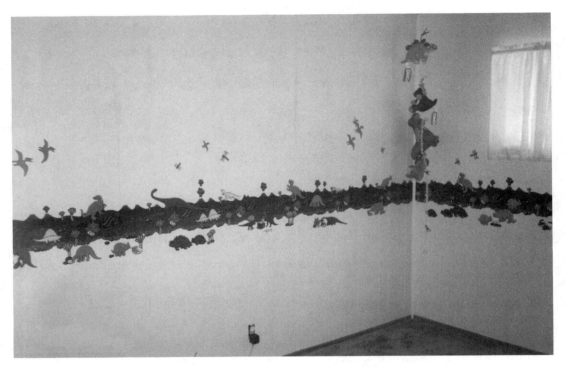

I took nesting to the fullest degree! I put up borders, mobiles, and a crib full of stuffed animals, bumper, and bedding.

## Wallpaper

Most wallpaper is made of vinyl, which is a plastic that has been treated with a variety of chemicals, including phenol and formaldehyde—not a good choice. These chemicals and plastics are not a good room addition if you are trying to create a toxin-free environment. The glue or adhesive used to seal the paper to the wall can be especially toxic; now you have a chemical mixed with more chemicals. See how easily chemicals add up in the room? And we are still talking about just the wall! There are safer, starch-based glues that can be used, but these may still contain unacceptable pesticides and fungus retardants. If there is toxic wallpaper in the room, consider removing it.

Borax (a water-soluble powdered mineral with antiseptic, antibacterial, and whitening properties; also called cetraborate and sodium borate) is often added to glues and adhesives to retard mold growth. Though borax is safe, the glue and adhesives are not. I have seen some newer products that are 90 percent recycled cotton, which give a kind of embossed look to the wall. This type of wallpaper has limited colors and textures, but it is a start. There are also more companies using Earth Paper, densely textured wallpaper made from paper pulp, stone powder, and straw with a water-based finish; it is another good option.

Manufacturers to look for at your local wall-covering store include Crown Corporation, Eurotap, and Pallas Textiles.

## Paint

Painting with a nontoxic paint is a less harmful option for decorating a room than using chemical-based wallpaper or paint. Faux finishing and stencils can add to the "look" without the toxins. If you are in a "Martha Stewart" mode, create your own stencil (you can buy them too) and use nontoxic paints to design your own motif. Again, be thoughtful when creating your sleep area, the place where your body rejuvenates itself from the day: Having toxic wallpaper and glue is a silent chemical attack on your body.

Several companies, such as Glidden, offer nontoxic paints and those with lower VOCs. These paints can be found in most places where paints are sold. AFM is another line of nontoxic paints, but you need to order it from The Living Source catalog (800-662-8787). When I decided to redecorate David's room, he and I decided on an animal motif, as he loves animals and nature. An artist friend used nontoxic paints to paint an animal and jungle mural on his walls. The result is stunning, one of a kind, and, most of all, safe. (See appendix for more sources of safe paints, Earth Paper, wall-covering, etc.)

## Good, Better, Best:  **Wall Coverings**

**Good:**    Be aware of toxic wall coverings in your home. Improve the air circulation (see "Air Quality," page 17).

**Better:**  Remove toxic wall coverings from sleeping areas.

**Best:**    Remove all toxic wall coverings throughout the house and replace with nontoxic paint. Stenciling and faux finishes can be used for accents.

## Better Choice Mom Recommends

*Earth Paper:* a densely textured, stuccolike wallpaper made from paper pulp, stone powder, and straw with a water-based finish

*recycled cotton wallpaper:* nontoxic wallpaper featuring an embossed texture; it can be ordered from Crown Corporation (see appendix) and Eurotap

For information on wall coverings such as indoor plywood and paneling, refer to *Your Home, Your Health and Well-Being,* by David Rousseau, W. J. Read, M.D., and Jean Enwright.

# *Carpeting*

There are two basic problems with most rugs and carpets and all wall-to-wall carpeting. First, they are toxic themselves. Second, they attract and hold on to more toxins, dirt, and dust. But not to worry for those of you who like something warm under your feet. You do have some options! But wall-to-wall, I have to be honest, is just not a good choice in your home.

Carpeting is potentially the biggest source of chemical outgassing in your house. Here is a list of chemicals that may be in your carpeting: 4-phenylcyclohexene (4-PC), 12-propylbenzene, 2-butyloctanol-1, 1,3,5-cclohlpatriene, 1,2,3-trimethylbenzene, 1-*H*-indene, acetone, azulene, benzene, bis(2-thylhxyl)phthalate, butadiene, caprolactam, decane, diethylene glycol, diisocyanate, thylybenzene, formaldehyde, hexane, styrene, toluene, vinylcyclohexene, xylene, and undecane-2,6-dimethyl.

These chemicals are added so that the carpeting is mold resistant, stain resistant, and moth repellant. Some of these chemicals are neurotoxins (damaging to the brain and nervous system), mutagenic (causing alteration of chromosomes or genes), carcinogenic, and/or respiratory irritants. And there's more!

This doesn't even take into consideration the toxic chemicals in the padding and the adhesive used to install carpeting. Are you beginning to get the idea? Altogether, your carpet could be outgassing over 100 chemicals. As a general rule, if you smell it, it is toxic. But even after it no longer smells, it can still be outgassing.

When doing my research, I was astounded by the tremendous number of registered health complaints regarding carpeting. Even the Environmental Protection Agency had to evacuate employees and remove 27,000 square feet of toxic carpeting from its own offices because of employee illness and complaints.

The health effects from everyday exposure to carpeting can be acute or chronic, and you may not realize what is happening. Reactions to carpeting have included headache, nausea, vomiting, asthma, respiratory problems, learning and memory problems, and even seizures. Do not expect doctors or other people to understand your concern about carpeting since many doctors are not trained about or do not believe in environmental illnesses/multiple chemical sensitivities.

In my case, it seemed to me that doctors thought I was just an "overreacting first-time mom" when I showed them the skin rashes, bumps, and swollen welts on David's body. I later discovered that all the chemicals in the wall-to-wall carpeting, the area rugs, and even the bath mat were contributing to David's eczema and sensitive skin. It was especially obvious after he had been sitting on the carpet. When he got up, his legs would be reddened with irritated skin. He would then begin to itch and start scratching.

Other children exhibit symptoms to carpet different from David's. For instance, I personally know many other mothers who've been told that their child's symptoms are just a cold or the flu; the mothers have later been able to establish a link between their child's symptoms and carpeting through observation, journaling, and trying different types of floor coverings.

Do not expect the carpet companies or manufacturers to understand your concern either. Their purpose is to make money; however, there are several companies aware of the issues that make safer carpeting. It is wise to get a sample of the carpet first and test it. You can have it tested for outgassing chemicals through Anderson Laboratories (see appendix, Toxin Testing). If cost is a factor, you can test it yourself by placing a sample under your pillow and seeing if there is a change in your sleep pattern or if you awaken with any symptoms.

This was a great test for my family. When we decided that we wanted our family room carpeted, I sent away for a sample of a highly recommended, high-grade carpet and placed it under David's pillow for a night. In the morning, his eyes were swollen, his nose was stopped up, and he had a dry, scratchy cough. Talk about mother's guilt! I can't imagine what David would have been like if we had gone ahead and installed the carpet without testing it first. (We ended up installing hardwood floors and purchased all-natural 100% organic rugs.) If you are intent on having carpeting in your home, testing a sample can save you a lot of money and possibly a lot of sleepless nights.

One common question with carpeting is, Can I treat the carpeting so the chemicals are no longer active? The answer is no. Many people are ill advised by carpet installers who recommend simply opening the windows or running the fan on your central air or heating for a while to get rid of toxic fumes. Running a fan is ineffective since carpeting is saturated with chemicals. In addition, carpeting can outgas for 20 years or more! However, if you do not have the option of removing existing carpeting, running a fan is better than doing nothing. People whose illnesses were due to carpeting found, however, that the only solution was to have it removed.

If you are absolutely not going to remove the carpeting, then ozonation with increased ventilation for a period of time while you are out of the house may cut down on outgassing. (Refer to "Air Filtration," page 20.)

In addition to the chemical problem, carpeting accumulates dust, mold, and animal dander, especially if you allow people to walk on it with shoes. Make people take their shoes off when they enter your house. (Japanese culture has always had a tradition of changing into *uwabaki,* or indoor shoes. To reinforce this, I give slippers as gifts to family and friends all the time.)

Leaving shoes at the door can be tough for family members if they are used to walking right on in. It can be a hard habit to break, but by persevering you save your family from an amazing amount of toxic garbage that gets tracked into the house by shoes. The toxins tracked in include weed killer or pesticides from lawns, dirt, mold, urine, feces, bacteria, and who knows what else. Studies have shown higher levels of pesticides, chemicals, and bacteria in the carpeting in homes where people wear their outdoor shoes inside.

Any way you look at it, carpeting is just not the ideal flooring. The least toxic floorings available are tile, true linoleum (made from linseed oil, pine tree resins, wood flour, and cork mixed with chalk clay and colored mineral pigments on a jute backing), and hardwood. With hardwood, make sure that the wood is not chemically treated and that you use safe adhesives and sealants or use the self-locking type that doesn't require adhesive.

I realize how expensive removing carpeting can be. It also takes proper planning to make such a dramatic change in your home and in your pocketbook, but this step alone can have the greatest impact on the air quality in your home. It took several years before I was able to afford to get rid of all the carpeting in our house. I tackled one room at a time, beginning in the bedroom since that was where we were inhaling the toxins while we slept, and then from there to the other rooms in order of their priority and use. I was fortunate that I didn't have carpeting in the kitchen, but I did have to deal with synthetic linoleum. I chose to give up some luxuries in order to make a healthier home, but I can tell you that it was worth the adjustment. I found that purchasing 100 percent cotton or chenille dhurrie (a flat, woven nonpile rug) and rag area rugs (instead of synthetic fiber carpets) allowed me to make my floors inviting—without all the toxins. (Area rugs still can attract dust and bacteria, so be sure to clean them as needed.)

---

### Good, Better, Best: **Carpeting**

**Good:**   Vacuum more frequently, get an air purifier, and do not wear outdoor shoes in the house.

**Better:**   Buy safer, healthier carpeting and padding with lower VOCs. Purchase 100 percent cotton or chenille dhurrie and rag rugs instead of synthetic fiber carpets to warm up your home.

**Best:**   Get rid of carpeting. Replace with tile, true linoleum, or hardwood.

Wash all area rugs in temperatures of 133 degrees Fahrenheit (56 degrees Celsius) or above to kill dust mites. Wool rugs can be dry-steam-cleaned at most dry cleaner facilities if you specify that method instead of traditional dry cleaning.

---

# Dust Control

I've been lucky to have the opportunity to travel and meet many of my Soapworks customers. Among the women I've met, not a single one likes to dust. Many times we put dusting at the bottom of our chore list because we think that "a little dust isn't that bad." Wrong.

Dust is not harmless. It can contribute to allergies, respiratory irritation, wheezing, sinus congestion, frequent colds, fatigue, and more. When I learned that 80 percent of house dust contains mites (microscopic creatures that live off dead skin) and small particles that have been shed from fabrics, soil, furniture, and animals, I had a whole new attitude toward dust. Dusting became a priority.

The house dust mite, *Dermatophagoides pteronyssinus,* is about half the size of a dot or period on a newspaper. The mite has no eyes and no organized breathing system, cannot drink, and lives for approximately three to four months. The mite may produce 20 droppings a day, which means approximately 2,000 droppings during its lifetime. The dust mite can get nourishment from its own droppings and may eat them up to three times over. (This is bad, but it gets more disgusting!)

Droppings are the main problem with dust mites. Dung pellets, if disturbed by activity, are pushed into the air. If this happens in an unventilated room, they can remain suspended in the still air to be breathed in by unsuspecting people—an invisible soup of dirt. It takes approximately 20 minutes for this "dust" to settle. Dust mites on their own are not a danger unless you're allergic to the protein in their fecal droppings. Certain individuals experience allergic reactions, such as asthma, rhinitis (hay fever), and some types of eczema.

Dust mites live off dead skin and the water vapor from our perspiration and breath, which is why they love our beds. If you are one of those people who hardly ever wash their bedding, think again! Though I do the laundry regularly, I wanted more protection for my family from these bugs, so I bought all-cotton barrier cloth encasements for the bedding and pillows to keep those nasty critters out! (See appendix for information.)

The humidity and temperature of the house contribute to the level of dust mites in your home. Higher humidity encourages the proliferation of dust mites as well as the growth of mold and fungus.

Ideally, humidity should be kept at about 40 to 50 percent or below to inhibit mites, mold, and fungus. You can purchase in most hardware stores a digital hydrothermometer that measures both humidity and temperature. Dehumidifiers help you take humidity out of the air. Dust mites thrive at a temperature of 77 degrees Fahrenheit, so if you keep the temperature lower than that, you'll reduce their reproduction.

When you are combating dust, it is important to remember that the cure must not be worse than the disease. If you begin your quest for dust control by shopping in catalogs that claim they sell hypoallergenic products, be aware that many products recommended to control dust mites in such catalogs are toxic. Do not solve one problem with another one.

Dust can be reduced by controlling what comes into your house, ridding the home of knickknacks, and dusting and vacuuming regularly. The type of furnishings in the room can also make a difference. A leather couch is preferable to a couch that has stuffed pillows (not to mention the Scotchgard that you might be inhaling!). In my home I got rid of all the miniblinds. They catch all the dust from inside the house as well as street dirt if they are in front of an open window. Dry dusting is practically useless because it just redistributes the dust. Aerosol dusting products are toxic and unnecessary. Either dust with a wet cloth or, better yet, use your vacuum cleaner. Most good vacuum cleaners (see page 41) come with a dust attachment that sucks the dust directly into the vacuum cleaner bag.

The best thing I did to control dust was upgrading the central heat and air-conditioning air filters, bringing in the air purification units for individual rooms, eliminating clutter, and making a commitment to dust thoroughly and regularly. These measures have reduced my son's asthma attacks.

## Good, Better, Best:  **Dust Control**

**Good:**   Be aware that dust in your home contains dust mites, animal dander, dirt particles, and toxins. Take shoes off when entering the house. Vacuum frequently with a quality vacuum. Wash all bedding at least once a week in water that is at least 130 degrees Fahrenheit. Avoid too many stuffed animals and clutter in rooms.

**Better:**   Buy all-cotton barrier cloth encasements for bedding and pillows to keep dust mites away from you when you sleep, which helps control dust mites throughout your home. Have the air ducts in your house professionally cleaned. Buy individual room air purifiers.

**Best:**   Avoid miniblinds and any other items that collect dust. Purchase leather-covered furniture since it avoids dust buildup. (Do not use toxic products to treat the leather.) Use all-cotton or all-linen lightweight curtains that have not been chemically treated and wash them regularly yourself. Deny the mites a home: Remove carpeting whenever possible. Install central or individual air purifiers. Keep temperature lower than 77 degrees Fahrenheit.

# *Vacuum Cleaners*

Did you know that when most of us are vacuuming, we're wasting our time? Many modern vacuums redistribute and stir up dust rather than getting rid of dust. Some studies that measure dust in the air show that there is more dust after vacuuming than before. This is due to poor design of the vacuum cleaner.

The purpose of a vacuum cleaner is to remove dust and dirt from carpeting, floors, furniture, and walls. If this is the case, tell me why a vacuum is upright. Isn't that going against gravity? Uprights have other problems as well. Most do not have powerful enough suction to adequately remove dust and particles from carpeting. Since they are not fully sealed to contain dust and do not have postmotor filtration, dust can escape. Lack of tight seals between components causes leaks. The fan or motor can actually spit dust right back out. This shows how poorly designed vacuums lead to more dust in the air after you vacuum.

Most uprights are practically useless for controlling dust. How many people actually cough, sneeze, and wheeze when they vacuum? This should not happen with a good-quality vacuum. The verdict? No matter how light and convenient an upright is, a canister vacuum gets the Better Choice Mom seal of approval!

Look for three things in a vacuum:

1. It must have powerful enough suction.

2. It must seal completely along the flow from where the dirt gets sucked into the bag to where the dust and dirt are stored. Watch your unit in the light and see if you see particles escaping. Feel around your unit to see if you feel air escaping.

3. It must have adequate filtration, HEPA being the most effective. HEPA filters microscopic particles down to .3 microns. In comparison, most vacuums remove particles down to only 35 microns.

One tested canister vacuum cleaner that produced cleaner air in the house after vacuuming is the Nilfisk. It is so efficient, it is used by NASA to eliminate microscopic particles from the cargo bay before any space shuttle leaves the ground. It is the standard to beat in terms of filtration.

The Miele Silver Moon with Power Brush is also another excellent HEPA vacuum with near-zero emission; however, it is a little more expensive than the Nilfisk. I had to save up to purchase the Miele vacuum, but it was well worth it for what it has done for our home. These are the top of the line, but there are several other HEPA filter vacuums that you can purchase.

Another option is a central vacuum, which is centrally installed in your home so that you take the hose from room to room and plug it into the wall where there is a latch. The main advantage to a central vacuum is that there is no chance that dust will be released back into the room since it is sucked into the wall. The bad news? Moving the 30-foot hose and attachments can be a heavy-duty task, and the unit is expensive to install. Some people swear by them, while others say they are very noisy and inconvenient and do not have the necessary suction.

Whatever kind of vacuum you choose, it is important to use and maintain it correctly. You should replace the bag when it is half to two-thirds full. If it gets too full, the airflow is reduced, and it loses suction capability, which means it cannot pick up the dust as well. You should also know how often to change the filters for the bag and the filter that protects the motor and be aware of other manufacturer recommendations. (See appendix for vacuums.)

## Good, Better, Best:  **Vacuuming**

**Good:**    Change the bag when half to two-thirds full. Maintain your vacuum properly. Vacuum often. Do not vacuum around things. Move and vacuum behind and under everything as well.

**Better:**  Replace upright with canister vacuum.

**Best:**    Invest in a high-quality HEPA vacuum.

# *Electromagnetic Fields*

Today not much is known about the health effects of electromagnetic fields (EMFs), but studies have shown that EMFs can affect human hormone levels and other important biological systems. They also seem to increase the toxicity of chemicals by allowing them more ready access to the sensitive nerve cells in the brain. (See page 249 for link to EMF research.)

Some very sensitive individuals are negatively and significantly affected by repeated exposure to energy produced from, among other things, microwaves, computer screens, and fluorescent lights. Man-made energy used for power and communication has totally changed the electromagnetic (energy) field in which we live. High-voltage power lines, transformers, cell phone towers, and television and radio antennas—anything that runs on electricity—all radiate EMFs. Now, most of us don't consider electricity a health hazard since it is just a normal part of modern life, but it's something to think about now that EMFs are beginning to be acknowledged as a health hazard.

Here are some of the concerns or claims regarding EMFs:

- chest pain, headaches, blurry vision, and any unexplained discomfort while sitting directly in front of a standard computer or TV

- mood changes, lowered immune system function, and learning disabilities

- a higher incidence of cancer among people living near high-voltage power lines, as reported in research from Sweden

- a possible link between cell phones and brain cancer

- a possible link between microwaves and brain tumors and genetic mutations

There are two basic types of power lines: transmission lines and distribution lines. *Transmission lines* are high-voltage power lines that carry power long distances from generator facilities to substations near urban areas. Substations contain transformers, which change the high voltage to lower voltages. *Distribution lines* then carry power from the substations to businesses and homes.

Each step of the way, EMFs are being transmitted around us 24 hours a day. No one wants to get rid of the modern conveniences, myself included, but you can make choices to eliminate toxins over which you do have control.

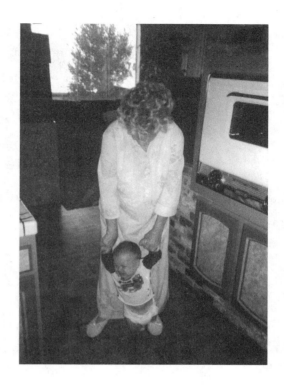

As if David doesn't have enough problems, Grandma is taking David for a walk right in front of the double ovens, and the heat from the oven is making the ammonia on the floor rise, adding to his distress.

Inside your house, anything that plugs into the wall—every electrical appliance—radiates an electromagnetic field. Again, I am not asking you to stop using your electricity, but I am suggesting you take an inventory on how much you have plugged in that you never use.

There are devices that measure EMFs and show how many EMFs your body is being exposed to and at what distance. This is good information. You can use it to help determine how far you should be from EMFs. Take the TV, for example. How close should you sit? When I was a little girl, my brother and I always sat close to the TV so we could easily change channels. Mom was a bit ahead of her time telling us to move back from the TV.

Of course, we don't need a gauge to realize that sitting six feet away from the TV is safer than right up on the screen, but what about computers? Many of us sit close to our monitors for much of the day. Again, information from a gauge may help you see what our bodies go through in one day just to fight off all the toxins.

Here's a general guideline for you: three feet from most electronic devices and six feet from the television.

## Good, Better, Best:　**EMFs**

**Good:**　Get rid of the bedroom TV and use a battery-operated alarm clock. Inventory how many things in your room are plugged in and then evaluate how many things from that list that you use on a daily basis. Unplug what you can.

**Better:**　Remove as many EMFs from your bedroom as possible and focus on the three feet around your head and sleeping area. Force yourself to commit to no more than two to four things plugged in per room. Install EMF devices so that you have a clear and accurate measure of how many EMFs your body is taking in every day.

**Best:**　Install a special electrical switch called a kill switch, which stops electrical emission from the outlet until the switch is turned on. This way you stop the current in the room when an appliance is not in use. Remove EMFs in your sleeping environment, especially those within three feet of your head. This includes wall outlets.

## Better Choice Mom Recommends

EMFs are a tough subject to cover. It was one of the last issues I tackled when redoing my house and continues to be one of my toughest issues. Many things in our modern society have to do with quicker, better, faster, and they all seem to have EMFs. I'm not suggesting you go back to living without electricity or the wonderful things that technology has provided for us. I am asking you to be aware of how much you overload your home and health. Give your family a "safe room" where there are few to no EMFs. I tried to create safe rooms in our bedrooms first and then worked my way out into other areas of my home. Trust me, David and I have had several long discussions over whether he can have a

TV, video games, and a telephone in his room—to all of which the answer is no. I have set up a room for David's video games and boom box, but it's not his bedroom.

You should choose what's best for you. The great thing is that you can continue to make changes and modifications over time. Rome was not built in a day.

The following Web sites are good sources of information on electromagnetic fields:

www.lessemf.com

www.fms-corp.com

www.promolife.com

www.aros.net

www.emf-bioshield.com

www.action-electronics.com

www.emf-meter.com

For more information, read *Cross Currents* by Robert Becker, M.D.

## Better Choice Mom Wisdom

As much as we moms would love to be outside, the reality is that most of us are relegated to indoor tasks, meaning that is where we spend 90 percent of our time. Studies show that stay-at-home moms have higher rates of cancer and other diseases than working moms. Scary! Why are we getting so sick? Many experts (you know, the ones with all the initials after their names), plus myself, believe that these new illnesses and almost epidemic increases in asthma are partially due to all the toxins in the home. This makes it *essential* for each of us to learn about the toxins around us, the health hazards they pose, and what we can do to reduce the risk to ourselves and our families.

Becoming more aware is half the battle. The other half is taking steps to change the toxic environment in our homes. I did my own home makeover step by step and day by day, making small changes and then moving on to bigger ones as I began to feel and see the results. Nothing needs to be done overnight. This book is meant to help you begin to see the potential sources of problems in your home and to help you make better choices for you and your children. You can take back control of how you and your family feel one choice at a time.

# CHAPTER 3

# The F.A.C.T.S. About Toxins in Your Home

It is our choices, Harry, that show who we are, far more than our abilities.
—J. K. Rowling, *Harry Potter and the Chamber of Secrets*

BEFORE DAVID WAS BORN, I never thought about reading a label, shopping for organic products, or even considering that some of the conveniences and luxuries that I took for granted and so enjoyed might be harmful. Who knew that so many chemicals were in these products that we so readily accepted in the name of progress? Toothpaste, milk, diet drinks, shampoos, and fast foods that we use on a daily basis are loaded with harmful toxins and chemicals. When David's illness became part of my life, I could take nothing for granted again.

From what I have learned from my research, David was not born sick. What happened was that he was more susceptible to toxins than some babies, and his sickness was compounded when he was overexposed to ammonia, a common ingredient in cleaning products. I cleaned with a vengeance; after all, I wanted my home spotless for my baby. These days, any amount of chemical exposure, from a heavy whiff of perfume to carpet freshener, can cause David breathing problems, such as an asthma attack, or skin rashes. Even the most unsuspecting things, such as clothes, sheets, and blankets, are, as I learned, saturated in formaldehyde to prevent wrinkling. (How many times do people come over to see your wrinkle-free sheets?) Something as innocent as getting Chinese takeout from a restaurant that uses monosodium glutamate (MSG) can trigger an asthma attack in David or alter his behavior from being quiet and playing nicely to being irritable, fidgety, or downright nasty. It was a relief, finally, to find a name for what David was suffering from: multiple chemical sensitivities (MCS). I finally knew I wasn't crazy, but I also recognized that "normalcy" was still a long way off.

The bad news is that most of the chemicals used in today's products are so well camouflaged that it would take a room full of experts to determine the true ingredients. If it is not a food product the law does not require the manufacturer to list all the ingredients. But I needed to know exactly what was in products because my son's welfare and quality of life depended on me knowing and understanding these toxins. How does an everyday mom who doesn't have a Harvard education or a chemistry background begin to unravel the mystery of what labels mean? I could not even pronounce the names of the ingredients or understand the acronyms (PEG, SLS), let alone figure out how they affected my son.

My first step was to look for the most common toxins in my home. That meant taking a closer look at everything, from the carpet and furniture to household products that I purchased. I had to ask what it was made of, whether the ingredients were synthetic or natural, how long the shelf life was—the questions went on and on. I recognized my lack of expertise in this area, so I researched even harder. I did hours of reading and asked hundreds of questions of experts, authors, and people who had children with similar challenges. My small progress gave me the confidence to continue until I got the answers. (At this point, I've been researching for nine years, and I'm still learning!)

Once I understood the side effects of chemicals—for example, formaldehyde can cause insomnia, and ammonia opens lung passageways—I was able to decide if a purchase was worth it. "Do I want to take the risk of David experiencing this side effect versus the benefit of what the product offers?" or "Is there a better choice that doesn't hold the possibility of a side effect?" I felt strong knowing I consciously was choosing what I used.

Once I began to dig deeper, I learned that there are a lot of different names for the same base chemicals. Do you know how many different ways alcohol can be listed in an ingredient list? Trust me, there are too many to memorize. I figured that if I couldn't even pronounce certain ingredients, then maybe I needed to ask more questions before I brought these ingredients into my home. I was drawn to products that used simple ingredients, such as water, baking soda, vinegar, corn syrup, and milk, but I stayed away from words that had 20 or more letters or that I could not understand. I also relied heavily on my journal for information on how David and I were feeling after I used a particular product.

After I figured out that these "mystery" ingredients might be harmful to David, the next step was trying to understand why manufacturers were using these toxins. What was their function or use in the product? (I couldn't substitute something for something else if I didn't know why it is was there in the first place.) Once I understood that natural ingredients cost much more than synthetic, toxic ingredients, it became obvious to me that the companies we trusted were using toxic components to make more money. Manufacturers use toxic chemicals such as formaldehyde in products, from fabric to food, to make them last up to 10 times longer, without regard for consumers' health.

Once I put a name to the toxins and figured out their use, I could then identify what products contained them, and I stood a better chance of waging a war on toxins and chemicals in my home. On my label-reading campaign, I soon learned that the most common toxins in our homes are these:

- formaldehyde

- ammonia

- chlorine

- tobacco smoke

- synthetic fragrances

It pains me that there are so many chemicals that infiltrate our homes, and to cover them all, this book would need to be volumes! However, to give you a platform from which to get started making your home toxin and chemical free, I felt it best to limit this discussion to the top five chemicals in our homes and products. These five toxins came up over and over again in my research. I truly believe, because I saw it for myself, that if you begin to remove these five toxins from your life, you'll begin to notice amazing changes in the way you think and feel.

Through my journal, I made the link that using products with these chemicals coincided with David's multiple chemical sensitivities (MCS) and asthma attacks. The answer, though not easy to find, was right there. I had to start eliminating these "toxic creeps" from my son's life and begin making better choices.

My next concern was to figure out a way to teach David how to recognize and stay away from these harmful toxins. Somehow I had to explain to him that, although playing in the plastic tubes at his favorite kids' pizza restaurant and switching lunches with his friends might seem harmless and a lot of fun, it could trigger a major asthma or MCS attack. Since no instruction book came with David's illness, I learned my lessons the hard way. After leaving several birthday parties to drive David, gasping for breath, to the hospital, I started to ask myself, why at birthday parties? What was the connection between the restaurant's play area and David not being able to breathe? In reviewing my journal, which I always carried with me, I saw that David's attacks always took place once he entered the plastic crawl tubes or immersed himself in the plastic balls. So I began to research

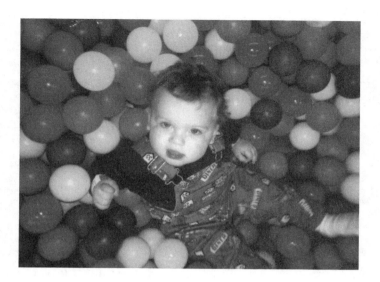

David should be having the time of his life in the plastic balls, but this fun day ended with him gasping for air and having a rash wherever the crawl tube and balls had touched his skin.

plastic. The information on plastic and what it does to your body made me downright ill, but I still wasn't convinced that the "bad guy" was the plastic. (See page 252 for Bill Moyer report, *Trade Secrets,* on plastics.) David's reaction, once in the tube, seemed too immediate, so I inquired about how the facility maintained the tubes: How were they cleaned since hundreds of kids used them every day? I found out that many other kid-friendly restaurants used chlorine to sanitize the play areas. Bingo; lightbulb! I already knew that ammonia was one of David's triggers, so I began to wonder if chlorine could be just as hazardous to his health. The information about chlorine's harmful side effects is positively overwhelming. Once I had read about the hazards of using chlorine and the number of symptoms it can cause, I knew what was making David so ill at these parties. Attending a simple birthday party was now a challenge in David's world. To add one more kick in my gut (do any children make it easy on their mom?), David thought that switching lunches and snacks on play dates and in preschool was fun. That ended quite abruptly when he found himself losing his lunch all over a classmate. Here I had spent hours deciding on the best snack and fun lunch, and all that effort was worthless the minute he traded it for a Twinkie. When I realized that he was beginning to make his own choices and beginning to be his own person, I knew my job of creating a healthier home was much bigger than just me getting information. I realized that I somehow needed to teach David so that he was well armed to face his challenges outside our four walls.

Since David was still very young, I came up with a game called F.A.C.T.S., which stands for formaldehyde, ammonia, chlorine, tobacco smoke, and synthetic fragrances. The game was an easy and fun way for him to remember these hidden toxins and feel empowered to avoid them. Before he sat down on a carpet, I would ask, "Are there F.A.C.T.S.?" and he would choose to pull over a chair instead of sitting on the carpeting. He learned simple rules, such as natural has little or no smell but toxins generally do smell, and a fragrance such as "lemon" might not exactly be fresh, let alone real citrus. David began to look at everything with a more discerning eye (not bad for a four-year-old!), asking himself if there were any F.A.C.T.S. in each item.

In order to create as "friendly" an environment for David as possible, I also had to teach my family, his teachers, friends, and neighbors about F.A.C.T.S. What happened was that not only did David begin to have a better understanding of his condition, but he also felt more understood by those who were an important part of his life. These people also benefited from this newfound knowledge. They too began to feel better as chronic health problems began to disappear. The changes we were making in our life were having a ripple effect, just as I hope this book will have for you and your loved ones.

## Toxic Creeps

Let's look more closely at the F.A.C.T.S., which are the most common toxins hiding in and around your home. There are too many household chemicals to cover in this chapter (there I go again with those scare tactics), so, again, we'll just stick to the most common five.

First lesson: When it comes to cleaning products, less is more. I can't tell you how many products I took out of my home that were half empty and shoved in the back of my cupboards. They had been abandoned mostly because they didn't work. Once I threw all those old products out, I had room for healthier products. Now it's your turn: Arm yourself with a sturdy cardboard box and begin removing toxic products from your home. (Remember to contact your local government for information on how to properly dispose of your toxins. Some cities have a pickup date for toxic materials, while others have a drop-off location.) Now the hunt for the F.A.C.T.S. in your house begins.

## Formaldehyde

Prior to my journey with David, the only association I had had with the word "formaldehyde" was the embalming fluid used to preserve frogs in my high school biology class. Never in my wildest dreams would I have looked for formaldehyde in my toothpaste and tampons. The scary thing is that, while we were not looking, someone made the decision to use this chemical everywhere—and I do mean everywhere—in our homes!

Formaldehyde is a preservative or binder that can be found in cosmetics, plastics, pesticides, cleaners, paints, waxes, polishes, mouthwash, and adhesives. It is also used in permanent-press fabrics. Now, when do you not use one of these items on a daily basis, and who would have known formaldehyde was in these products? Even if we had thought to look, we might not have found it because formaldehyde is a toxin that hides under many different names. In addition, there are by-products of formaldehyde to watch out for. Perhaps aspartame sounds familiar to those who drink diet sodas. Well, guess what? Aspartame is a by-product of formaldehyde! Yum, drink up!

One of the primary uses of formaldehyde is in the manufacturing of cabinets, flooring, walls, carpet, and furniture. Formaldehyde is also made into glues that are mixed with wood scraps and chips to produce particleboard, plywood, fiberboard, and other substitutes for solid wood. A good clue that formaldehyde might be hidden in the product is this: The cheaper the wood, the more likely that it is a wood "product" held together with formaldehyde. Virtually every American home built or renovated since World War II is full of this toxic creep.

Though there are many problems with formaldehyde, one that is a major concern is that it outgasses, a process in which toxic vapors are released from solid objects much as steam rises from hot water. We normally think of solid objects as being permanent, inactive, or inert, but this is not the case. Particleboard and other treated materials are constantly releasing toxic vapors into the air we breathe. Virtually everything synthetic or containing rubber or plastic outgasses formaldehyde and other chemicals. This is partially why it is believed that our indoor air is worse than the outdoor air, and perhaps this is why respiratory and breathing problems are on the rise.

Since the late 1970s, it has been known that formaldehyde causes cancer in rats, and it is now listed as a reasonably anticipated carcinogen. (The number of proven carcinogens is comparatively small, but many more chemicals are suspected to be carcinogenic. A partial list of known and suspected carcinogens is maintained at http://physchem.ox.ac.uk/MSDS/carcinogens.html). What does this mean? It means that it has been shown to kill animals. Many argue that there is not necessarily a correlation between what happens in animals and what happens in humans, but if this is the case, why is there animal testing at all? For me, the conclusion does not need further debate.

If you choose not to believe that formaldehyde is linked to cancer, however, there are sufficient other health problems associated

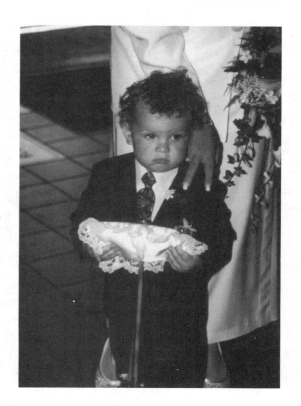

David, wearing a synthetic suit more than likely loaded with formaldehyde, was not a happy boy and was in discomfort as he walked down the aisle as a ring bearer.

with formaldehyde to raise concern. It can cause headaches, depression, dizziness, insomnia, asthma, heart palpitations, shortness of breath, bladder problems, and irritation to the eyes, nose, throat, lungs, and skin. It is hard to understand why such a toxic chemical is still being manufactured today.

Formaldehyde is also considered a strong sensitizer. This means that formaldehyde exposure could cause you to become sensitive to other chemicals that were not a problem prior to exposure to formaldehyde. I learned how this could change a person's life forever in watching this happen to my son, as described at the beginning of this chapter. Unfortunately, there is no guideline as to how much of an exposure can cause this type of sensitizing because everyone's body and immune system are different. It can come from one large exposure, such as the spraying of pesticides at school or home, or from chronic daily exposures to perfume, laundry detergent, or deodorant. If you know someone with chronic fatigue syndrome they will tell you that one day they were fine and the next day they called it quits. Studies have shown that the sickness has been linked to constant bombardment of toxins. This is downright scary when it comes to children and their little, growing bodies.

The only way to truly control formaldehyde is to select materials that do not contain this ingredient. Especially toxic are cheap desks and book cabinets that you put together yourself. Though you may not be able to smell it, furniture can still be outgassing toxic chemicals, even when it is no longer new. If you cannot remove items containing formaldehyde, sometimes they can be treated or sealed with such products as Safe Coat or Crystal Air. There are companies that make natural products, including furniture, that are not treated with formaldehyde (see appendix for sources). A better choice is untreated solid wood, such as pine or oak.

If cabinets in your house that likely contain formaldehyde are 10 years old or older, they may have outgassed significantly already and may not be a large source of formaldehyde. Certain items, such as a school binder that comes complete with that all-new smell, will outgas only a short time and may not be problematic. You can speed up the process of outgassing by putting such items as a binder or new shower curtain in the hot sun for a few days to allow the smell to dissipate. There is no timetable that says when a product has completed outgassing. Again, whenever possible, avoid purchasing such items.

Another option to consider if you cannot get rid of items that are outgassing is to have your home treated with ozone. Ozone combines with formaldehyde and other volatile organic compounds and oxidizes them, transforming them into carbon dioxide and water.

There are companies that can come to your house and run an ozone generator. This is particularly effective for removing odors from fires as well as keeping down the levels of dust mites and bacteria. This treatment can be done only when the house is unoccupied.

You can buy air purifiers that emit ozone to use on a daily basis (see page 22). These obviously release much lower levels of ozone than the professional units. I have used them and now have switched to high-grade air purification units.

## Good, Better, Best: **Formaldehyde**

**Good:**    Become aware of sources of formaldehyde in your house, such as particleboard, linoleum, and Formica. Seal them with safe sealants. To prevent the release of more toxic vapors, do not clean formaldehyde-containing furniture or other items with corrosive cleaning products.

**Better:**    Buy furniture and other household furnishings that have been labeled as low-emission board, which has less formaldehyde. Check the manufacturer's information. Some will be stamped as exposure 1 or exterior classification, which indicates that less formaldehyde has been used.

**Best:**    Eliminate particleboard and other synthetic materials from the house. Avoid future purchases of this type. Buy natural materials, such as metal or wood, that are not treated with chemicals.

## Better Choice Mom Recommends

Formaldehyde is so abundant in so many products that it is beyond the scope of this book to list them all. There are entire books on the subject. See *The Poisoning of Our Homes and Workplaces: The Truth about the Indoor Formaldehyde Crisis* by Jack Trasher, Ph.D., and Alan Broughton, M.D.

## Ammonia

Grandma bought pure ammonia in a clearly labeled bottle and used it primarily for cleaning around the home. Now ammonia is hidden in so many products, from cleaning to personal care, that you do not even know when you are buying or using it. The big danger is that most people (me included, until I learned otherwise) do not know that ammonia is a powerful chemical and carries a high price. In David's case, the fumes from the ammonia burned the lining of his lungs, which caused his asthma, and burned his eyes. Today, even if he just brushes against a surface where a product that contained ammonia was used, he breaks out in a rash. This one ingredient caused David many sleepless nights, hours of painful scratching, and many trips to the hospital to help him breathe.

On its own, ammonia is dangerous, but when mixed with other chemicals, it can be deadly. Did you know this? Probably not! It is easy to accidentally mix ammonia with other chemicals because the labels on name-brand cleaning products neglect to inform the consumer as to what the active ingredients are.

I learned this the hard way when cleaning the bathroom. For years I cleaned the toilet with a scouring powder that contained bleach and used an ammonia-based window cleaner to polish the tank. The problem came when I mixed the two together. I almost knocked myself unconscious when I cleaned the toilet with both products at the same time. Little did I know that bleach and ammonia create a toxic bomb, commonly known as mustard gas or chloramines, which can cause choking, coughing, and lung damage.

Many products are a combination of different chemicals, and in many cases only half the truth is told on the labels as to how dangerous these products are when used incorrectly or in conjunction with others. As you can see from my experience, it is easy for accidents to happen.

There are actually two types of ammonia: natural ammonia and man-made ammonia. Natural ammonia is formed when manure, plants, and animals decompose. This type presents no health threat. Man-made ammonia, however, is toxic.

Household (man-made) ammonia contains 5 to 10 percent ammonia and releases fumes that are extremely irritating. Even low amounts can cause severe eye, lung, and skin irritation. Repeated exposures can damage the eyes, liver, and kidneys as well as cause bronchitis with cough, congestion, and shortness of breath. Children with asthma may be especially sensitive. For those of you who have kids with a dry cough, you may want to consider this connection.

Using ammonia without adequate ventilation makes any side effects worse and is more likely to cause a bad reaction. Accidental spills, skin contact, or swallowing ammonia is not uncommon in children and can have devastating effects, including the following:

- Eye contact can cause severe burns, cataracts, glaucoma, and even eye damage and blindness.

- Skin contact can cause burns and open sores if the area is not washed immediately.

- Swallowing ammonia can actually cause burns in the mouth, throat, and stomach.

- Breathing in concentrated ammonia fumes can cause symptoms ranging from headache, nausea, and vomiting to fluid buildup in the lungs, which is a medical emergency.

Avoiding these potential nightmares is easy. Get rid of cleaners that contain ammonia. If you don't know what is in a particular cleaner, out it goes! (See appendix for alternatives to oven and window cleaners.) Eliminating the use of ammonia products also benefits the environment since ammonia is one of the toxic chemicals most commonly dumped into our water supply. Remember, what you dump down the drain comes back to you in your drinking water. I cannot stress this enough: Do not dispose of these chemical-laden cleaners by dumping them down the drain. Please contact your city for proper disposal.

Other sources of ammonia, besides household cleaning products, to which your children may be exposed include cigarette smoke (contains traces of ammonia), fertilizers (if children play on grass or play at a park or on a sports field that was recently treated), waste sites and industrial spills in residential areas, and decaying manure (if you live near large farms where animals have been exposed to chemicals).

## Good, Better, Best:  **Ammonia**

**Good:**  Be aware of the products that contain ammonia (such as window cleaners, other cleaning products, deodorants, and disinfectants), and do not mix or store these products with other products that contain chemicals.

**Better:**  Limit your toxic supplies to two or three in the household. Store and use properly.

**Best:**  Choose products that use natural ingredients, such as citrus, instead of ammonia. The cleaning power is just as effective, without those harmful ingredients.

## Better Choice Mom Recommends

Try Soapworks or Seventh Generation brands of all-purpose household cleaners and Bon Ami for scouring powder.

## Chlorine

If you do nothing else with this chapter, please go get your bleach bottle and read the manufacturer's warnings. If the label from the people who make it is not enough proof for you that this chemical should absolutely not be in your home, perhaps the following will make you get rid of it now! In addition to its other health effects, chlorine can be devastating to pregnant women. Studies have linked chlorine and miscarriages.

According to Doris Rapp, M.D., in her book *Is This Your Child's World? How You Can Fix the Schools and Homes That Are Making Your Children Sick*, chlorine is the "C" in deadly PCB and the source of the "chloro" in chlorofluorocarbons, which degrade ozone. Chlorine is crucial in manufacturing many poisons, including Agent Orange (used to defoliate the jungles during the Vietnam War) and DDT. Rapp says, "Dioxin, a by-product of the industrial use of chlorine, is considered by many scientists to be the deadliest chemical ever made. It has been linked to cancer, miscarriages, birth defects, reduced sperm counts and learning disabilities." This is a scary chemical.

Using chlorine bleach is one of the most harmful and unnecessary practices in this country, yet the product is still sold in stores throughout the United States. Chlorine-containing chemicals are persistent, or bioaccumulate, which means they do not break down easily but accumulate in the environment and in our bodies. As a result, the environmental effects of chlorine are disastrous, as are the health effects.

Chlorine is an irritant and a corrosive. It can irritate the lungs and respiratory passages if inhaled. On contact, chlorine can burn the skin, eyes, and other membranes. When I saw the X rays of my son's lungs and the burned facile (small hairs in the lungs), I had all the proof I needed that chlorine and ammonia were poisoning my child. The X rays revealed the reaction of David's small, not-yet-developed body and immune system to the chlorine and ammonia hidden in my everyday cleaning products. (Since children are still growing, their bodies are like sponges, able to have a greater absorption rate than adults.)

These products were sold to me under the "all-American, suitable for your entire family" label, which led me to believe they were safe and gave me no clue about the potentially dire consequences of using them. Even just washing David's clothes with laundry detergent containing chlorine bleach caused numerous skin problems and asthma attacks before I made the connection. (It was the residue left on his clothes.) Also, David was constantly diagnosed with "prickly heat." I have now learned that he didn't suffer from prickly heat at all; the red, swollen bumps that covered his body were his skin's reaction to chlorine. When I began to look at him with a more discerning eye, I noticed that the parts of his body not covered or touched by clothes had little or no rash. I've been able to duplicate the reaction numerous times by stripping him of all clothes and "airing him out." No diaper, no clothes, no rash. (No wonder I have so many photos of a naked baby David!) But when I put a sock on him, his foot and ankle would break out in bumps. After speaking to many moms over the years, I find that a common diagnosis from doctors when they see little red bumps is prickly heat, or hives, which get treated with a steroid or ointment. In reality, there are many causes for the skin to react with bumps. The cure is eliminating the cause so there is nothing to treat.

Though not everyone reacts the same way to chlorine, chlorine-sensitive individuals should not go in swimming pools or hot tubs that contain chlorine. Indoors, they need to have a filter installed centrally for the whole house, which would include drinking water from the faucet and at the shower and tub. If their clothes are washed with bleach, some individuals break out in a rash, especially when doing athletic activities, which cause the pores to open, giving the chlorine access into the body. Children, who tend to have more

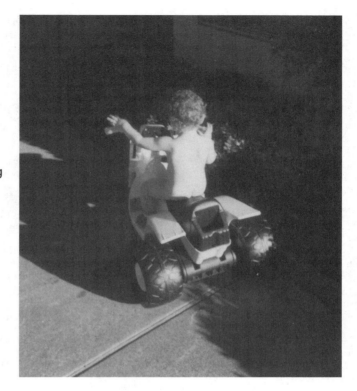

David was so much more comfortable without clothing that on his third birthday, there he was riding his new motorcycle in the buff!

sensitive skin than adults, may get a rash on their legs or ankles from the top of their socks or on the skin in contact with the elasticized bands of their underwear. Unfortunately, these rashes are often misdiagnosed, so we lather our children with medicated creams and throw out a brand new pair of socks. Isn't that like throwing out the baby with the bathwater?

As a result of all these dangers and health problems, some scientists are now saying there are no safe, allowable limits for chlorine. In fact, in 1994, the EPA called for a complete ban on its use (as part of its Clean Water Plan), but large chemical manufacturers, as you can imagine, mounted a countercampaign. Still, some corporate giants have done the responsible thing and are offering safe, effective alternatives to chlorine. For example, one major fast-food chain is phasing out its chlorine-bleached french-fry bags, many copy stores are offering "chlorine-free" bleached paper, and commercial manufacturers now sell laundry detergents with "bleach alternative." (Bleach is the same as liquid chlorine but half as strong.)

## Good, Better, Best:  **Chlorine**

**Good:**    Know if you have chlorine products in your house and store them separate from other cleaning products.

**Better:**    Use chlorine bleach sparingly in washing clothes and only on items you feel you must, such as socks that were worn outside. (Okay, your husband's workout clothes, if you insist.) Wash hands thoroughly after any contact. Double rinse your laundry.

**Best:**    Avoid coming into contact with chlorine. Buy nonchlorine bleach for laundry and non-bleached paper products, tampons, toilet paper, and napkins. Use natural cleansers or homemade recipes for everyday jobs and purchase nonchlorine bleach for laundering your whites and colors.

(See appendix for recipes for homemade cleansers.)

## Better Choice Mom Recommends

Try Soapworks Non-Chlorine Bleach, Oxi-Clean, or Ecover Non-Chlorine Bleach. Try Seventh Generation and Green Forest brands for nonbleached paper goods.

## Tobacco Smoke

More than enough has been said about the hazards of cigarette smoking and secondhand smoke. This is an issue that I fight every day. Simply eating in a restaurant where smoke has no boundaries and can easily creep into the nonsmoking section can trigger an asthma attack in David.

More and more places are not allowing smoking, and I have been fortunate that most people have been when considerate. I always tell smokers that I am happy to move but please "give us a minute" so we can leave. Most people have been kind enough to put out the cigarette. I have no right to ask someone to stop, so it is my responsibility to remove myself from the situation.

No, I am not going to start a crusade to get you to stop smoking, but it is one of the best gifts you can give your children. Tell them you did it for them.

---

### Good, Better, Best: **Smoking**

**Good:**   abstinence

**Better:**   abstinence

**Best:**   abstinence

---

## Synthetic Fragrances

Who would have thought that the rose scent in your candle came from a factory, not from a lovely rose garden? You may think a product that is touted as having a "natural lemon or lavender scent" gets that scent from a plant, but more than likely its odor was manufactured in a laboratory. The word "fragrance" in cosmetics, personal care products, and cleaning products can refer to any one of 4,000 different ingredients, most of which are synthetic, none of which come from flowers!

The source of the fragrance can be a combination of numerous ingredients; however, you will rarely find those listed on the label (label reading again). Many of these synthetic compounds are carcinogenic or toxic to the body and produce adverse reactions such as rashes or other allergic symptoms. Many times it is the synthetic fragrance in a product that causes a reaction rather than the product itself.

A much safer alternative is to buy unscented products and add your own essential oils, though some people cannot even tolerate oils. If that is the case, they should use only unscented products.

Switching from synthetic fragrances to pure essential oils often allows people to enjoy a wonderful variety of scents in the home. Another benefit of essential oils is that they are naturally antiseptic and fungicidal.

**Properties of Essential Oils**

- antibacterial, antiviral, antifungal, antiparasitic, and antiseptic
- stimulate the immune system
- increase oxygen, negative ions, and ozone
- provide a delivery system for nutrients directly to cells
- assimilate into the body in 25 minutes without leaving any residues

Essential oils are not all equal in quality, so when purchasing them, you need to know which are high-quality or pure oil. There are three grades of essential oils: grade A (therapeutic), B (food grade), and C (perfume grade). Over 90 percent of the essential oils in this country are of the lower grades and are less expensive and of poor quality. Most of those oils are cut with other oils, alcohol, chemicals, or synthetics that can cause them to go rancid.

Therapeutic grade is the highest quality, purest, and, yes, most expensive. This means if you bought a small bottle of an essential oil at a health food store for $5, it is probably not the quality needed for the best results. Don't be misled by a claim of "100 percent natural." Most retailers sell one of the lower grades that have been adulterated by being cut or diluted with odorless or potentially toxic solvents. Of imported essential oils, less than 3 percent are therapeutic grade.

## Good, Better, Best: **Fragrance**

**Good:** Limit the number of synthetically fragranced products you purchase and bring into your home.

**Better:** Buy products that use essential oils rather than synthetics.

**Best:** Go all natural. It really is not that hard to do with the many new companies that offer all-natural products. By supporting these companies, you're sending the message that the hidden toxins are unacceptable.

## Better Choice Mom Recommends

To get high-quality essential oils, you may have to find a source on the Internet or an independent distributor. One good product is Top of the Mountain Essential Oils (www.thetopofthemountain.com). The National Association of Holistic Aromatherapy is a nonprofit organization that has a listing of essential oil distributors at www.naha.org.

## Better Choice Mom Wisdom

Every day we are faced with choices, from what we choose to drink to what shampoos we use and what food we eat. Now that you've become more aware of the hazards contained in even everyday products and have learned about safe alternatives, you're in a position to make better choices. There are products that can "do their job," that is, clean your hair, quench your thirst, or decorate your home, without being harmful to you, your family, and the environment.

As I mentioned before, the list of chemicals covered in this chapter is in no way complete. As you become an avid label reader, as I have, you'll become more familiar with what "lies within" your purchases.

# CHAPTER 4

# The Kitchen

## Would You Cook Dinner in Your Bedroom?

Every person has free choice. Free to obey or disobey the Natural Laws. Your choice determines the consequences. Nobody ever did, or ever will, escape the consequences of his choices.
—Alfred A. Montapert

THE KITCHEN IS BY FAR my favorite room in the house. Perhaps it's because of the many hours I spent there cooking with my mom or the times grandma was preparing a sauce for Sunday dinner while I was discussing my latest interests. It was hard for me to believe that this "sacred place," full of wonderful smells and delicious food, a room that brought me such warmth and happiness, turned out to be my greatest challenge to rid of chemicals and make it an organized and functional room. It was a room of contradictions: How could this place that I always loved now be a harmful environment?

The bad memories for me about the kitchen are that it was the room where I first discovered what was causing David to be so sick, and it was the place of some of his agonizing screams. The good memories are that the kitchen was also the room where Soapworks was born, which totally changed my son's life and my own for the better.

As with most families, many of life's activities when I was growing up seemed to happen in the kitchen. We cooked in the kitchen, pressed clothes, sorted laundry, did homework, paid bills, and had numerous projects going on at the kitchen table. My own playpen was in the kitchen so mom could keep an eye on me. My toys (pots and pans) were on the floor to keep me busy while she cooked. At night my father and friends would play cards at the table while the women talked about the kids, school, and whatever else was happening.

Since this picture was so clear in my head, I carried most of these same habits into my own home when I had David. In fact, on the first day I brought him home from the hospital, I set his baby carrier on the kitchen table as family and friends gathered to see the new arrival. Ironically, when I look back, it was as early as that day that his painful crying started.

Though being in the kitchen that day was the trigger for David's condition, I didn't put it all together or truly understand David's challenge until he was almost a year old. It was over this period of time that I learned about and began to understand all the issues that can lead to a less-than-healthy household and life.

The kitchen will probably always remain to many of us the heart of the home, and it is still the room where I spend a great deal of my time. But, here comes the bad news again, though it is all about warmth, happiness, and fond memories, it is also the room that harbors some of our greatest dangers.

To begin the process of making better choices for your kitchen, I ask that you acknowledge what you want to happen, not what happens, in the kitchen. When it comes to making good, better, and best choices for you and your family, you need to ask the questions, "Is this room the best place for all these other activities?" and "Is the purpose of the room—cooking—being diffused and made less efficient because of these other activities?" In other words, can you really do what needs to be done in the kitchen with all of those other things going on, taking up space and cluttering the task at hand?

There is no way to distinguish the good from the bad if you cannot see what's happening in a room—how would you know you need to organize?

Once I saw the chaos of the kitchen more clearly through my journaling, I was able to reorganize the space so that it accommodates tasks and activities more effectively. Once I defined the room's purpose, I began looking at all the things that did not belong, which led me to understand why my grandma always said to "keep things simple." One set of silverware is more than sufficient, so why mix and match three sets? Why have 13 coffee mugs (you *know* there are some with chips and others discolored so badly you are not even sure what color they were) when you use only 5 of them regularly? It was hard in the beginning to toss out things that were "still good," even though they were rarely used. I really didn't need a toaster because I already owned a toaster oven, which has the same function. I had a container filled with spoons and spatulas, but I used the same two all the time. Why have dozens? Once I got into the "pitching and tossing" mode, it felt like a weight was lifted. I began to see my kitchen clearly—and finally to see where there were problems. And boy, were there problems!

Once I did detective work through keeping my journal, it was obvious that there were some definite links/causes to David's challenges, particularly with his breathing and his skin rashes (eczema). I saw a clear pattern: After I cleaned his high chair, baby swing, playpen, carrying car seat, bouncer, and other items using an ammonia-based counter cleanser before David used them, he would start to change almost immediately. What happened was that David ended up not being able to breathe, his skin swelled with red welts, and he would have a huge temper tantrum. Even his arms would break out in the areas where he was leaning on the tray. I was just

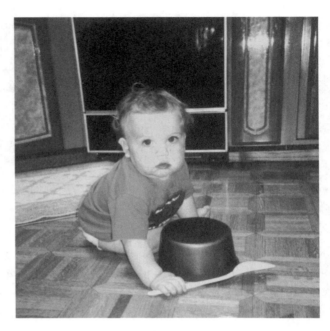

David doing what he loved to do—
be with me in the kitchen
and play with his "toys."

trying to keep his environment clean, but the residue from the cleanser was aggravating his skin. I also used to put him on the floor to play with his toys. One thing he loved was playing on the floor with my food containers, which I kept in a bottom drawer. Once again from the journal, I saw the same symptoms as when he was in his high chair or on other places I had cleaned. It was then I realized that I cleaned the hardwood floors with bleach and ammonia and that the food containers he was playing with were plastic. Unknowingly, I was poisoning my child by doing things that I had seen and learned from my mother and almost every other mother I knew!

When I stopped cleaning with ammonia, put tile on my floor, and put David on an all-cotton rug when he was playing at my feet, his physical symptoms disappeared, as did the temper tantrums. The aroma in my kitchen before I began keeping a journal was what I thought was a "clean" smell. What I really was smelling was chemicals. What you smell now in my kitchen is nothing.

The kitchen is one of the busiest rooms in the house. Because of that, it is important to record any activity that happens in this room, not just the ones that have to do with cooking and eating. To make this process easy, make a list of the things you already know go on in the kitchen, including the time that they occur. Time is important because the purpose of the room may change as the day unfolds. Leave room in the list for unexpected things. Enter activities and times as they occur. Once you move through this process, you will be surprised at how many different things go on in the kitchen in one day.

As an example, here's my kitchen in the morning: David and I always have breakfast together, just the two of us, which is one of our special bonding times (I pack his lunches and lay out his backpack at night). My girlfriend's morning kitchen "assignment," on the other hand, is completely different. For her, it is making lunches and locating backpacks and finding car keys and generally getting her family off for the day. Her kitchen functions differently than mine, so it needs to be re-created and organized to suit her needs.

## Journal Questions: Kitchen

### Questions to help locate toxins

1. Can I identify and see everything under my kitchen sink without moving anything, or is it cluttered?

2. Do I keep vitamins and medicines in the kitchen? How many of them have expired?

3. Do I have multiple products for the same purpose in the cabinets, such as countertop cleaners, window cleaners, and oven cleaners?

4. How many of the exact same products do I have?

5. Have I bought economy-size items but have no room for storage so that they get placed here and there? Am I able to use all the product before its expiration date?

6. Am I storing highly toxic products like drain cleaners, oven cleaners, and automatic dish detergent in an area that is easy to reach as well as next to one another? Is there anyone in my home who could get his or her hands on them who could be at risk?

7. Do I have cross ventilation in this room, meaning is there a way to get air to flow in and out of both sides of the room?

8. Where does the air from my exhaust fan in the kitchen go? Out of the house, into the attic, or into another room?

## Questions to help organize

1. What would I like my focus to be in the kitchen? Cooking? Family gathering place?

2. Can I see the tops of my counters, or are they covered with appliances, papers, notes, and car keys?

3. Are things easily found by me as well as others?

4. Are there stacks of papers that I have no idea what they are or their purpose?

5. Do I throw out a lot of spoiled food?

6. Do I buy a food item, a new utensil, or a paper product only to find I already had one hidden away?

7. What is my mood when I walk into the kitchen? Happy? Overwhelmed?

8. Do I have a feeling of stagnation in my kitchen? Just one "honey do" list after another?

9. Do I enjoy my time in the kitchen?

10. Do I have everything I need there, or am I constantly going to another room?

11. Is the kitchen organized in a way that supports the purpose I have defined for this room?

12. Does the kitchen have the necessary "inspiration" or motivational elements for its purpose?

13. Is it time to get rid of old appliances and treat myself to one I have been wanting for a while?

■ ■ ■

During the journal process or when it is completed, it should be apparent what you really do in the kitchen. You will discover that other tasks are harder to do in the kitchen when it is set up for cooking and eating and not for other activities. You'll see what is efficient and what is not, what you want to remove and what you want to add. The journal process will truly help you define the purpose of this room and set up the parameters for its makeover.

Make sure to involve the whole family in redefining and redesigning the kitchen so that everyone's thoughts and ideas are incorporated. If you include everyone in your family in this "defining process," it will cut down on the whining later. Of course, if you are a control freak or consider this room your domain, then you will have to deal with your issue of letting go.

Because David really enjoys cooking (I wonder where he gets that from?), he often likes to invite his friends over to eat. Since our kitchen is now redesigned around cooking and entertaining—all the other activities of our lives have their proper place—having a bunch of nine-year-olds in my kitchen is much less chaotic than it would be if I were still trying to do my bills on the countertop.

The following are issues to consider in redesigning the kitchen:

■ organization

■ cabinets

- countertops

- flooring

- ventilation and air quality

- appliances

- food preparation and storage

- cleaning

- kitchen pest control

## *Organization*

If you're like many of us, the first thing that may jump out at you is that there is way too much stuff in your kitchen. Whether it is all kitchen paraphernalia or not, it is probably still too much. So in your journal, write down what you have in the kitchen and then highlight what really needs to be there, keeping in mind the purpose of the kitchen, which you determined with your journal. Take a cold, hard look at your inventory and decide if there is anything that can go either to another room or to the garbage.

You might want to try what I did and see what you discover. I took my food processor, coffeemaker, coffee grinder (I am not a coffee drinker but kept the pot, grinder, and beans on the counter for friends), and mixer and moved them into the garage to see if I would miss them. The funny thing is that I've used them once since I reorganized. Those items were just taking up space. I have the same chopper that I have used for years and never really found the need to use the food processor. I find that I use the same cooking spoon, pot, and pan time after time. When redoing the kitchen, I made the items that I used regularly easy to get to and moved the "expendables," such as dishes I seldom use, into an area designed for storage.

A reminder, though: Be sure to wash stored items before you use them since just by sitting, they can accumulate fumes, oil, grease, and dust.

Again and again I try to show people how clutter slows them down and distracts them from their focus. One thing that I've found is that most successful people have little or no clutter in their homes. You will begin to notice in kitchens of people you admire that there is no "extra fluff" and that many small appliances, such as a juicer, a toaster, and a coffeemaker, are hidden from view. Ever wonder why? Focus! If you are focused, you accomplish things efficiently. (See Suggested Readings for Suze Orman's books *The Courage to Be Rich* and *Nine Steps to Financial Freedom.*) The idea here is to use it or lose it. If it is not being used, it is time for it to go elsewhere or even out! If you cannot see uncluttered space and open areas on your counters, then the space is not defined.

The final part of your kitchen inventory is to reorganize the kitchen drawers. Dump out the contents of your cabinets and drawers, take a look at what is there, ask yourself what you use, and then begin to organize or in some cases discard. Start by putting the necessary ("necessary" being the key word here) and like items in the same place. By creating a baking drawer, kids' drawer, silverware drawer, and so forth, you are separating and defining for everyone in your family where something is and where it gets put back. Having this defined space cuts down on the endless "Mom, have you seen my . . . ?" cries from around the house.

To help in this process, purchase drawer organizers to separate paring knives from spatulas, utensils from eggbeaters. (See appendix for stores.) A common issue for many of us is holding on to old silverware. I cannot tell you how many people have a drawer full of old, mismatched, dull knives (dull knives are actually more dangerous than sharp ones; since you have to use more force, you have less control) and bent forks. This is enough to frustrate anyone, let alone make setting the table a less-than-desirable chore. Do not buy new "anything" without getting rid of the old. That is not progress. If you cannot bear to throw something away, donate it. If you cannot even do that, box it up (with a label, please) and get it out of the kitchen.

Many of us learned from our moms the way to arrange a kitchen: pots, pans, baking dishes, and assorted cookware on the bottom shelves; dishes near the dishwasher; a baking cupboard; a seasoning cupboard; and similar food items stored together, that is, pasta with pasta and all the canned goods in one place. Though this appears to be a good and functional plan, it is not the only way to do it; in fact, there is no right or wrong way. Since everybody in the household uses the kitchen, how it functions and how it is organized is key to the success of your healthy makeover.

### clutter + chaos = dust = bacteria and germs

What will become clear to you from your journal is this: How the kitchen should be organized depends on the people who are using it.

What I've done in my home is to create designated areas in the kitchen for each person's "things," both personal things and kitchen things. If you choose to organize this way, then each member of your family should have his or her own cupboard, shelf in the pantry, or defined counter space. For instance, David has his own supply of foods he likes, his plates and utensils, and even his own cookware in his area. He loves to come home from school and make fresh juices. If I want him to make the juice, then the juicer needs to be in a place easily accessible to him, as do the glass, utensils, fruit, yogurt, or anything else he might put into his smoothie or juice drink. His designated area also holds personal items, such as his bookbag, his lunch box, and an in basket for things he needs me to look at.

I haven't added pull-out drawers in my kitchen yet, but they are fabulous! You can easily see what's on the shelf, and they are easy to line with a nontoxic cloth or unbleached paper towel so you can easily clean with no hassle.

I have found it particularly interesting that, like my mother, I chose to put all the canned goods in one place. Now tell me, what does chicken stock have to do with tuna fish? I can't imagine David using broth, but I certainly can see him making a tuna fish sandwich.

Don't get me wrong: There are certainly drawers or cupboards where you need to put like items together, such as the everyday dishes and silverware. But even these decisions should be made with your whole family in mind. In my home, it is David's job to take the silverware out of the dishwasher and put it away. I would prefer that the silverware be near where I need it most, where I cook, but that is across the kitchen from the dishwasher. That is not the best place for David, who drops things along the way. So I moved the silverware drawer next to the dishwasher.

Organizing according to family members' uses also helped me lose weight. The food that my son eats, such as bread, muffins, cookies, and fruit juices, easily distracts me. Setting up my own cabinets with my no-yolk pasta and low-fat snacks and crackers gives me a safe place to look for something to eat. What I don't see I don't eat—most of the time!

This method also goes for organizing the food in the refrigerator. We may expect a five-year-old to make his own chocolate milk, yet we keep the milk on a top shelf, and, even worse, it is in a gallon container. Now that is an accident waiting to happen! My grand-mother always kept a small creamer of milk in the refrigerator, ready to pour on her cereal or in her tea. Today, David and I have carried on that tradition. A small creamer is easy to handle; milk is easy to pour; it takes only seconds to refill; and if it is left out, there is little waste. I can't remember ever having an accident with spilled milk in my home. I think grandma was on to something.

Make sure all of your children's foods are in child-friendly con-tainers and in places that make it easy for them to "self-serve." When I did this, I found David made better food choices. Since there are so many chemicals in foods, he is never tempted to grab something that may be harmful to him because I don't keep those items in "his" area.

If you take this new approach to organization, you'll make your kitchen a more efficient and organized place and—as we'll discuss later in the chapter—a healthier environment as well. The icing on the cake is that you've taught your child some independence! This means mom doesn't have to jump up every time her kids need something. They begin to learn to do it themselves, mom has made her life easier, and we have begun grooming responsible adults.

## Good, Better, Best:  **Organization**

**Good:**    Organize around what you use, not what you have.

**Better:**    Define spaces for each person who uses the kitchen.

**Best:**    Remove everything that is not being used.

## Better Choice Mom Recommends

Here are some great hints.

- Transfer kid items—juice, milk, cereal—to kid-size containers.
- Introduce your children to their areas—drawer, shelf, and cupboard—so they can find and maintain what is theirs.
- Store your glasses upside down to keep out dust, germs, and bacteria. This also forces you to grab the glass from the bottom instead of the top, keeping fingers off the part where you drink.
- Store cutting boards vertically and put them away after using so they dry.
- Oil your wooden utensils, cutting boards, and salad bowls with olive or vegetable oil to keep the wood from drying out, which extends their life.

# *Cabinets*

Cabinets are absolutely essential for keeping our lives organized and functioning. They are where we store our food, glassware, and dishes. Unfortunately, the majority of the building materials used to make cabinets can cause some health risks. Let's discuss what your cabinets are made of and how you use them.

Most cabinets made in the past 20 years are constructed from particleboard, which, as you know from previous chapters, contains formaldehyde and different kinds of toxic glue. Since the kitchen is usually the hottest room in the house and heat releases toxins, the cabinets are producing poisonous gas at a fast and steady rate. And this is where we keep the food?

No need to panic; there are definitely some great alternatives that are cost effective and aesthetically pleasing. Remember, when I first learned about all these potential health hazards, remodeling a kitchen was not in the budget, so I had to get creative in finding out the best ways to work within my means. I began by sealing the cabinets (see appendix) and using a nontoxic, noncorrosive product to clean them. This way, abrasive cleaner was not eating into the particleboard and releasing chemicals into my cabinets and into the air. I used, and still do, a cotton sheet cut to size to line the cabinets. That way, when the liner gets dirty, I just wash it and return it to the cabinet. You can also use all-natural paper towels and toss them when they get soiled.

If you're storing your dishes in cabinets near a heat source, guess what? If you've used toxic dishwashing detergent to clean the dishes, the heat will reactivate the toxic residue on the dishes. Also, even food items that recommend "store at room temperature" can be affected by a nearby heat source; the quality of the food might be reduced or, worse yet, the structure of the food might change. Food items can spoil quicker if exposed to heat.

For those who can afford it, I recommend replacing your wood-like cabinets with real wood; or if you can't replace them, take off the door and use glass doors, a popular look today taken from the 1940s. Both are healthier choices and a great alternative to the heavy look of wood.

---

## Good, Better, Best: **Cabinets**

**Good:** Organize your cabinets so that susceptible foodstuffs and the dishes you use most often are in the cabinets farthest from the heat sources (oven, stove, and refrigerator).

**Better:** Use a nontoxic sealant, paint, or stain on the cabinets. Clean them with a nonabrasive, natural all-purpose cleanser. Replace fabricated wood doors with glass.

**Best:** Replace the particleboard cabinets with cabinets made of solid wood. This means the frames as well as the fronts.

---

# *Countertops*

Choosing the material for your kitchen countertops is one of the most important decisions you can make toward having a healthy home. Think about how often you use your counter. Take it one step further. Think about how often your food comes in direct contact with the counter. And think about how often our hands come in contact with the counter, after which we put them near or on our own or our child's face.

Unfortunately, most builders use less expensive but oh-so-toxic materials, so replacing the countertops needs to be added to your "to do eventually" list. I'm a big fan of natural materials—marble, granite, clay, ceramic, wood. Butcher-block counters are quite popular, as well as functional and attractive. Tile is great, too, though you have to be careful about what is in the grout and in the grout sealer.

Also, remember, with tile, the bigger the tile, the better. Smaller tiles require more grout, which increases exposure to substances that can cause some people to have a skin, respiratory, or behavior reaction. (Children as well as adults can get grouchy from exposure to toxins.) If you are able to choose the countertops for your kitchen, make your decision three-dimensional, not just about what looks great. For instance, if you choose granite, investigate the frame the granite sits on. What is it made of (it might be particleboard), and what attaches the countertops to the cabinets (make sure it is nontoxic glue)? Finally, when you've put this beautiful natural material in your kitchen, don't create another health problem by cleaning it with a toxic chemical. Use a gentle, natural cleanser.

If you are like the majority of us, you have laminate countertops. Not only does laminate sit on a particleboard frame, but what makes laminate? You got it—formaldehyde. You may not be in a position to replace the countertops, so what do you do today to protect your family? Clean wisely. Here is why: If you have a countertop that contains formaldehyde and you use a corrosive, aggressive, dirt-eating product, the chlorine or other chemicals in the cleanser eat through the top sealer, releasing the formaldehyde. The laminate countertop is already outgassing, but you have just increased the output. You don't need such a cleaner; it is overkill. Use a gentle, natural cleaner instead. Ingredients such as citrus (lemon) and grapeseed extract are natural antiseptics. (See appendix for cleaning recipes and alternative products.) They cut grease and kill germs without the dangers of toxic chemicals.

If changing neither your countertops nor your cleaning product works for you, at least be aware of what your countertops might be adding to your food. Do not place your food directly on the countertop; set it on a paper towel. Make your sandwich on a plate or cutting board. (If you are making lunch for the next day's meal, do not go to all this effort of health-wise preparation and then stick the sandwich in a plastic bag.)

## Good, Better, Best: **Countertops**

**Good:**    Keep food off the countertop by placing it on a plate, napkin, or wooden cutting board.

**Better:**    Still keep food off the countertop and use a natural cleaner that does not corrode the countertop.

**Best:**    Choose a natural countertop material, such as stone, granite, marble, tile, or wood and clean with an all-natural cleaner.

## Better Choice Mom Recommends

Get rid of your kitchen sponge! It is a breeding ground for germs, bacteria, and your basic yuck! Use 100 percent cotton washrags, a mere $2.99 for a bag of 25 that can be thrown into the laundry at the end of the day. Or purchase paper towels. Seventh Generation and Green Forest paper products are made from unbleached and recycled paper.

# *Flooring*

It used to be that the only choice you had for a kitchen floor was laminate, and you can imagine how I feel about that! Just as with the countertops and the particleboard (from which the subfloor is probably made), the formaldehyde and other toxins used to make the flooring continually outgas and do so even more when it is warm. And what happens when you cook? The kitchen heats up! Feel the floor around the refrigerator. It's hot. What happens under the dishwasher? It gets hot, too. And what does hot air do? It rises. Having laminate flooring in the kitchen is just like having poisonous gases rising from a toxic swamp. And this is where we let our children play?

Carpeting is also an absolute no-no in the kitchen. Aside from the chemicals in the carpet, it is a storage place for dust, mold, bacteria, and particles of food.

Fortunately, today there are many natural options for flooring that are aesthetically pleasing and reasonably priced. Stone, marble, tile (remember, bigger squares are better), and hardwood floors are excellent options. Warning: Do not use the synthetic hardwoods. Guess what? They are just laminate stuck together with chemicals and made to look like wood, and they put you just as much at risk as vinyl or laminate.

If you are not able to change the floor in your kitchen, treat the surface with respect. If you know you have a loaded gun, you carry it differently than if you know the gun is not loaded. The loaded gun is the toxic floor in your kitchen. Just as with your countertops, do not use a corrosive cleaning agent. If you do, you are slowly peeling off the top layer and releasing toxins into the air. A gentle, natural cleaner or an all-purpose cleaner can be used on flooring. You do not need an extra special, strong cleaner. Again, it is overkill. If you are standing in the kitchen or the baby plays on the floor, put a barrier between the toxins and you and your baby by placing an all-natural blanket or rug down on the floor.

Bleach is the worst. Some people like to add a little to the cleaning water because they want the floor to be sterile. I understand the concern, especially with younger kids crawling on the floor, but the immediate fumes from the bleach are toxic and they linger and corrode the floor. And the other real big issue is, do you know what you are mixing together? Children who crawl and play on the floor not only smell the fumes more closely than we do in a standing position but also get the residue all over their hands, which we know will end up in their mouth and on their clothes. This was one reason David had sores in and around his mouth.

So instead of bleach, try one of the many natural antibacterial, antimicrobial essential oils and safe cleaning products. They work, and they don't poison you!

## Good, Better, Best:  **Flooring**

**Good:**　Put a barrier, such as a cotton rug, between you or your child and the surface if the surface is a laminate or carpeting.

**Better:**　Clean with nonabrasive cleaners.

**Best:**　Replace the floor with stone, marble, natural wood, or tile.

## Better Choice Mom Recommends

If you're concerned about having a sterile floor, use hydrogen peroxide or citruses like lemons, grapefruit, lime, and oranges. Better yet, try grapeseed extract. (See appendix for cleaning recipes.)

# *Ventilation and Air Quality*

Nowhere in the house is ventilation more important than in the kitchen. Most kitchens are not designed with enough ventilation. Cooking produces odors that you don't necessarily want, but at least the odors are not dangerous. Cooking on a coil or with gas can be harmful and in some cases can cause a reaction if mixed with the outgassing from flooring, cabinets, countertops, and appliances. This makes your kitchen a potentially dangerous environment for adults and children.

For stoves, the most efficient and quiet ventilators have remote blowers, with the blower and motor attached to an outside wall and connected to the stove via a metal duct. This way the air is blown outside, not simply recirculated throughout the house. When running a ventilator, you also need a source of intake air. Opening a window in the kitchen is sufficient.

Even though my home is new, I had this problem because my exhaust went into my attic. I had an appliance repairman redirect my exhaust fan to the outside of our home and had one of the nonopening windows converted into an opening window. I also put an air purifier in my kitchen. This made a huge change in ridding the kitchen of odors; with the air purifier, cooking fish is not such a chore. The purifier also cuts down on dust and helps keep the air clean overall.

## Good, Better, Best: **Ventilation and Air Quality**

**Good:**    Create cross ventilation if you can.

**Better:**  Have an exhaust or air purifying system installed.

**Best:**    Have access to fresh air and recirculate air that has been filtered. Get rid of toxic items.

# Appliances

Any good designer will tell you that you can never have enough outlets in the kitchen. Think of all the things that need to be plugged in. First there are the major appliances: refrigerator, stove, oven, and dishwasher. Then there are all the smaller appliances: coffeemaker, toaster, microwave, mixer, juicer, and so on. All these small appliances create clutter (which is visually unappealing), electromagnetic fields (EMFs), and potential fire hazards. It is best to unplug small appliances when not in use. If the power goes out or you have a power surge, the appliance can be damaged or spark, which can start a fire. If you have enough space, I suggest storing the small appliances when not in use. If you can't or don't want to do that, you can purchase pretty coverings that go over the appliance. This also prevents dust accumulation. If your appliances are quite old, you may want to consider purchasing new ones. Many new appliances feature enhancements such as quieter motors and fewer EMFs. (See chapter 2.)

## Stove/Oven

Environmental medical specialists have found that the number one household hazard for environmentally sensitive people is a gas range. After removing gas stoves from the house, many people found immediate relief from chronic symptoms. If you are not going to replace your gas range or are unable to, you should understand the risks and how to maintain your gas range safely.

Natural gas is colorless, odorless, and tasteless. The gas company adds a chemical, mercaptan, which gives the gas an egglike smell to help in detecting gas leaks. Unfortunately, all people do not have the same sensitivity to the smell. If you have chronic allergies or a cold, you may not smell anything when there is a leak, and weather can also affect the strength of the smell. For these reasons, many times leaks go undetected. The pilot light goes out and you don't realize it. It is surprising how often this can occur, so if you have a gas stove, you need to be aware of the symptoms of natural gas poisoning. They are similar to those of carbon monoxide poisoning but are often confused with symptoms of the flu: weakness, headaches, fatigue, dizziness, visual problems, and difficulty thinking. Symptoms can vary with exposure:

- mild exposure: headache, nausea, and fatigue
- moderate exposure: severe throbbing headache, drowsiness, confusion, vomiting, and increased heart rate
- extreme exposure: unconsciousness, convulsions, cardiac or respiratory failure, and even death

Natural gas exposure in pregnant women has been linked to birth defects. Chronic low-grade exposure in children can lead to neurological disorders, memory loss, personality changes, and mild to severe forms of brain damage. Children are especially vulnerable to natural gas leaks because they have a higher metabolic rate and are more quickly affected by gas buildup and oxygen depletion.

Gas leaks aren't the only problem with gas stoves. Extended use (during holidays, for instance) without enough ventilation can also cause health problems because of oxygen depletion and buildup of combustion by-products: carbon monoxide and nitrogen dioxide. (We always wondered why grandma's eyes sparkled and she seemed a little loopy at holiday time. We thought she might be nipping at the wine, but maybe she was light-headed from the gas!)

You can purchase natural gas detectors at any home improvement store, which will alert you to leaks. Install one for each of your household gas appliances—stove, water heater, fireplace, and gas dryer. I have read one too many stories about people getting sick or dying from gas leaks in the home.

Electric ranges are much safer. There are no combustion by-products, and you also have the benefit of being able to have a lot of ventilation without disturbing flames. You do not have to worry about pilot lights going out or, worse yet, an open flame on the range top that can easily start a fire. Even though some cooks, myself included, say electric ranges are not as easy to cook with because of lack of temperature control, my thought is that the increased safety far outweighs that benefit—and I love to cook!

### Cleaning the Oven

Look at any oven cleaner, and you will probably find a strongly worded warning: "Do not breathe spray mist. Protect floor and all nearby surfaces with newspaper." It is the last precaution that really gets me. If I have to cover the area surrounding the oven from oven cleaner, why would I put it in the oven to begin with? It just doesn't seem possible that if you put cleaner in your oven, no matter how well you wipe it out (which means you are breathing it and touching it and otherwise doing everything the product label warns against), some of it, even just a little bit, won't still be there when you put food into the oven. In my world, even a little bit is too much.

My strategy is to control, as much as possible, the drips and spills in the oven so that I don't have to clean with a toxic agent. I put foil or an oven liner on the bottom, and on each of the racks I put a sheet of aluminum foil. The air is still able to circulate, but when drips fall on the foil I can just take out the dirty foil and replace it.

When you do need to clean the racks, I recommend using just hot water and a scrub brush. You might need to soak the rack for a while to get the really baked-on stuff off, but that is all it should take. Using good old-fashioned soap (all natural), vinegar, and hot water works, or I use my Soapworks all-purpose spray and liquid soap. For the hard, cooked-on food drips, borax mixed with water does the trick. To clean the inside of the oven, wipe with a cloth rag (not a sponge) and use the same products that you used on the racks. The oven will sparkle until the next spill!

## Dishwasher

A dishwasher is a wonderful thing, a great time and energy saver. Don't assume, however, that it is killing all the germs on your dishes, glasses, and utensils. Fortunately, there are things you can do to make your dishwasher an ally in your battle for a healthier home.

People rarely read appliance manuals to learn how to properly operate and maintain their appliances. Most manuals give helpful hints for maximizing an appliance's effectiveness. For instance, when I was reading my dishwasher manual, I learned that I should turn on the hot water at the sink tap until it is hot and *then* run the dishwasher. This fills the dishwasher with hot water when you turn it on. If your dishwasher fills with cold water, then it never hits the proper temperature for disinfecting. I've noticed a significant difference in my dishes since I started this simple habit. Newer dishwashers have options such as a water heat booster, which raises the temperature 20 to 50 degrees. Most people also do not know how to properly load the dishes. They develop bad habits, such as putting dishes covered with gobs of food into the machine and then letting them sit there for hours or even days before running the dishwasher. Gross! It is an invitation for bacteria and a good way to clog your drain. Here are some tips on getting the most out of your dishwasher:

1. Rinse the dishes first. If you have a garbage disposal, you can rinse food scraps off at the sink. If not, scrape the food into the garbage. This avoids clogging the drain in the dishwasher.

2. Load the dishwasher properly. Put small dishes in the middle, progressing from there to largest dishes on the outside. Putting larger dishes in the middle prevents the water from hitting the other dishes.

3. Place silverware in the basket with the handles pointing up. This way the water will hit the dirty part first.

4. Never put plastic in the dishwasher. Plastic releases chemical vapors under the heat. (Plus, if you use the booster as mentioned above, your plastic will melt.)

5. Never put wood in the dishwasher. The water and detergent not only ruin the wood but get trapped inside the wood and can create mold. Rinse wood with very hot water and rub it with a brush and maybe a little soap. Detergent dries out the wood, but real soap does not. Dry it, then wipe with a little olive, peanut, or vegetable oil.

6. Do not overload the machine. If you do, you'll end up with only partially clean dishes.

7. Before turning on the dishwasher, turn on the hot water at the sink tap and let it run until it is hot. This will ensure that the water running into the dishwasher will be hot enough to kill bacteria.

### Dishwasher Detergent

Have you ever noticed a funny taste when you drink from a glass just out of the dishwasher? Ever fill up a glass with water and see bubbles? Those bubbles are the leftover toxic residue from your dishwasher detergent. The manufacturers are nice enough to warn you on the package that the product is "harmful if swallowed," but if the detergent is still on the glasses when they are supposedly clean, how do you avoid swallowing it?

Over the past seven years, I have had many people complain to me about stomachaches and bad tastes in their mouths. Personally, I did not realize until after I switched dishwasher products that the product I had been using for years aggravated my ulcers. I created a Soapworks dishwasher product for this very reason. If you are reluctant to switch to a toxin-free dishwashing soap, at least rinse the dishes thoroughly. You can run the dishwasher rinse cycle twice or rinse them by hand. If detergent specks are left on the dishes after the cycle ends or it is not cleaning as well as you would like, it may be that not enough water is getting into the machine. The water inlet valve may need replacing; this needs to be done every five to six years.

So what is in dishwasher detergent anyway? Most mainstream detergents contain a lot of chlorine, sodium, and synthetic fragrance. And we are washing our dishes with this? What did we learn from chapter 3? Yum! The lovely smell you get when you open up the dishwasher after it has been run is from the chemicals that your machine did not wash away. Now put a sandwich on a plate and have lunch. Guess what went into your stomach with the sandwich? When you heat food on your dishes, you reactivate the detergent chemicals left behind, and they are absorbed right into your food.

A few years ago, gel detergent showed up on the grocery store shelves. What we did not consider when we bought it was that the dishwasher soap dispersal system was not designed to accommodate gels, so by using them we were actually limiting the efficiency of our dishwashers.

The half of the detergent cup that closes is designed to open when the dishwasher reaches 190 degrees. If you put a gel in the cup and turn on your dishwasher, the gel runs out of the closed cup. When the second cleaning cycle begins, the cup pops open and it is empty. The detergent is gone when it is time to clean and sanitize the dishes. The only way to correct this is to rinse the dishes thoroughly before you put them in the dishwasher. This way, the first cycle in the dishwasher becomes your second wash since you took the time to do the first wash by hand. In essence, the dishwasher has not washed the dishes, but it has sanitized them with the hot water. My conclusion on gels is, good-bye convenience, hello more work.

The other issue is cost. Gels stick and cake to the inside of the bottle, so you never get the last drop, meaning you get less product, which means you get fewer loads. Gels also cost more. So all around you are creating more work, it's costing you more, and it is potentially a health risk. Whose idea was it to come up with a gel? My suggestion is to stick to a nontoxic dishwashing powder. You alleviate the waste problem, the inefficient cleaning, and the toxic residue left on your dishes from standard dishwashing detergents.

## Better Choice Mom Recommends

Never put a wooden cutting board into the dishwasher. Clean it with natural soap and water and sanitize it with lemon juice. Before buying a toxic spot remover, consider using a vinegar and baking soda rinse placed in the dishwashing soap dish.

## Refrigerator

I will say it here: I hate cleaning out the refrigerator. But what I dislike even more is opening a fridge and seeing a science experiment! I hate the leftovers that have been marinating for weeks and are now uniden-tifiable, the veggies that have gone from crisp to soggy, and then the real surprises: what has fallen behind the drawers and under the glass!

If you want to rid your refrigerator and freezer of these great un-knowns, start by reorganizing so that when you open the door you know exactly what is in there. It may even help those people in your home who open the refrigerator door, stand there for an hour, and claim they cannot find the mayo that is staring at them. (Then again, it may not!)

I find that designating certain areas in the refrigerator for certain foods is ideal. This includes a spot for each member of your family, as I explained earlier in reference to the cabinets. Make it a general rule that you be able to see immediately what is in every container or pack-age. If you can't see it, use labels. This way, without opening the con-tainer, you can tell the leftover spaghetti sauce from the leftover gravy.

If you can't see everything in the refrigerator without rooting around, my guess is you have too much in there. A refrigerator needs air circulation to work properly anyway, so if it is packed, it cannot do its job. Why not do an inventory to see what you might be able to get rid of, put in a different spot, or store more efficiently? How many choices of jelly are really necessary? How many types of mustard do you really need? And when it comes to salad dressing, is yours one of the majority of homes that are on "salad dressing overload"? I observe a rule of never offering more than two choices of anything. I like to keep life simple. For those leftovers, we have a "must go" night every week. On Thursday, I take out every leftover in the refrigerator, any vegetables that may not make it until the weekend, and anything else that *must go,* and out of all this I create dinner. My son thought we were eating French food ("Must go" sounds like a foreign word to him), but he quickly caught on!

Another way to increase the efficiency of your refrigerator and make it healthier for your home is to make sure it is positioned correctly. A common mistake is to suffocate the refrigerator by placing it too closely to the wall or cabinets. A sure sign is when the wall behind the refrigerator is black. Most refrigerators eject heat from the bottom and/or back. There must be enough space to allow air to circulate and to dispense the heat. The amount of space needed varies from unit to unit, but use at least, if not double, the manufacturer's recommendation, which is usually four to six inches. Also, do not store anything next to the refrigerator, such as a stepping stool or paper bags or other things that might slip nicely into that space. Remember—breathing space.

These days we have more choices than ever in refrigerators—side-by-side, top freezer, or bottom freezer. Some are very energy efficient and have all kinds of bells and whistles—drink dispenser, ice crusher, and snack door. My advice is that you think carefully about the needs and abilities of your family and choose the refrigerator that will work best for everyone over time. For instance, if you have small children and you want to encourage them to be independent, a freezer on the bottom is probably not a good option because it puts items such as juice and milk up too high. Side-by-side allows your kids to get at every part of the unit, but then again, you may not want them going through the freezer, so a top freezer is a good option in that case. I purchased a refrigerator with an icemaker in the door right before David was born. Wrong! What a great game for David and his friends to see ice cubes come flying out!

I love the refrigerator drawers that have recently come on the market. They fit into the cabinets and look as if they are a cabinet yet are a refrigerated bin. They were originally designed as produce keepers, but I think they are great for kids' juices and other foods. The drawers are smaller, so they have less suction and are easier for little kids to open. It also means that your kids are not opening and closing the big fridge all the time, which makes the fridge more efficient.

### Cleaning the Refrigerator

Spills in the refrigerator are inevitable, but there is a way to combat them without having to clean your entire refrigerator. I place paper towels in all the bins and on all the shelves. When something spills, the towel absorbs much of it so it does not run all over. Then I just gather up the paper towel and replace it with another one. But this is for spills. You do have to give your refrigerator a thorough cleaning once in a while. When taking on this task (and this one can be a chore, I will admit), you want to avoid spraying a toxic cleaner on one shelf and then closing the door and trapping the chemicals inside with all the food. I recommend taking the shelf out of the refrigerator, cleaning it with a nontoxic product, letting it dry thoroughly, and then returning it.

I also line the top of my refrigerator with paper towels to combat the dust and grime that accumulate. Whether you keep things up there or not, dirt can gather and eventually get into the refrigerator or freezer every time you open the door.

## Better Choice Mom Recommends

How do you make yourself an efficient refrigerator user?

- Offer only two choices of condiments.

- Store food in see-through or labeled containers so foods can be identified quickly.

- Designate shelf space in the refrigerator for each member of your family so they know where to look for their items and where to put them back.

- Use paper towels as bin and shelf liners.

- No stacking!

## Good, Better, Best: **Appliances**

**Good:** Understand how the manufacturer recommends you use the appliance—read the manual!

**Better:** Routinely clean your disposal, dishwasher, washing machine, and garbage disposal with vinegar and baking soda rinses.

**Best:** Purchase energy-efficient appliances that suit your family's needs.

# *Food Preparation and Storage*

The makeover for the kitchen has to include how you prepare and store your food. We can unwittingly create health problems if this is not done correctly.

## Food Preparation

Not only do you need to be a smart food shopper, you need to know how to treat your food once you bring it into the home. If you have taken the time to purchase natural food but then make the food on a countertop just sprayed with a toxic cleaner, why bother with the natural food? Or you buy tofu, wrap it up in plastic, and microwave. I believe wooden cutting boards are a must if you have countertops of synthetic material. Wooden spoons are preferable to plastic. In other words, play the F.A.C.T.S. game (chapter 3) with yourself when preparing food. After a while it will become second nature.

### *Microwaves*

The convenience and speed of using a microwave oven for cooking are seductive, but there are two important health questions to consider:

(1) Is this the best cooking method for maintaining the nutrient value of our food, and (2) what kind of radiation exposure are we getting from the appliance when using it and eating food from it?

In answer to the first question, some of the potential dangers from microwaving food are the following:

- decreased nutrient value compared to some cooking methods
- leaching of packaging or plastics into food
- the potential formation of carcinogenic substances in the food

Aside from what it does to the food, the radiation emitted when the microwave is running is a real concern. Children love to stand in front of it and watch the food being cooked. This is a "never, ever" for both children and adults!

If the door or hinges are damaged, radiation leaks. And since you can't see radiation with your eyes, you won't know it's leaking. Manufacturers' manuals and consumer advocate groups advise that you have your microwave checked annually for leaks by a qualified repairperson. But where do you even find such a person? And such a service call would probably be more expensive than what you paid for the microwave in the first place. To be on the safe side, you can purchase a microwave oven leak detector at a minimal cost and check it yourself. Look for these devices in your local hardware stores and appliance shops.

## Better Choice Mom Recommends

The following Web sites provide further information about safety in the home. Some also offer safe products for the house.

www.safetyhero.com

www.comforthouse.com

www.ccrane.com

www.professionalequipment.com

## Food Storage

How many products come in plastic? If at all possible, store products like cereal, pasta, lunch meat, and so forth in glass containers. The manufacturer's box doesn't keep your $5.00 box of cereal fresh anyway. If you don't have glass containers, lining your plastic storage containers with a paper towel is a good start.

Purchase a 20-piece set of glass storage containers in lieu of the traditional 20-piece plastic set available at discount stores. If you cannot live without unbreakable plastic containers, another option is to wrap the food in wax paper. Obviously, this is not for liquid food. (Refer to Bill Moyer report on plastics, "Trade Secrets.")

When possible, remove food from store packaging and store in airtight glass jars because toxins can't penetrate glass. In addition, plastic breathes, allowing air in, which oxidizes the food so it spoils more quickly than it does when stored in glass.

**air + food = spoilage**

**light + bread = mold**

A habit to avoid is coming home from a restaurant and storing leftovers in the restaurant's Styrofoam container. When you do this, the food absorbs the chemicals from the Styrofoam, which you can tell by the plasticlike taste you get when you eat the food the next day. A bad situation is made worse by microwaving the Styrofoam container. Never, never, I say, never, put food in the microwave while it is in plastic or Styrofoam. This includes plastic wrap and bags. Heat increases the release of chemicals from the plastic, and they go right into your food.

A good habit to get into is to put your restaurant leftovers into an ovenproof glass container as soon as you get home. Then they are ready to be reheated. Reheating in a toaster oven, the oven, or a steamer is best. It may take five more minutes than heating in a microwave, but you won't get any radiation.

## Better Choice Mom Recommends

Keep these stocked in your kitchen:

- wax paper baggies

- Butter Bell (a round ceramic cylinder that stores your butter in one-quarter inch of water; found in upscale kitchen stores)

# *Cleaning*

With the growing demand for nontoxic products, more and more companies are making products without harmful chemicals. Part of my commitment in learning how to make soap and other products was to bring them to the shelves for you. But you don't have to buy my products. You can do most of your cleaning chores in the home just like Grandma did—and do them safely. Here are the must-haves for a natural, nontoxic home. Remember, what you choose to clean with comes into contact with your family either through breathing it, touching it, or eating it.

- *White vinegar.* Good for cleaning shower doors, tubs, and sinks. Use equal parts warm water and white vinegar in a spray bottle and use as you would any all-purpose spray. Great for shower curtains and windows.

- *Baking soda.* Great for making a paste (with white vinegar) to clean your stainless steel. Baking soda is also great for perspiration stains in your clothes. Make a paste of baking soda and water and let the paste soak on the stains for up to 30 minutes. Wash normally.

- *Lemon and lemon juice.* A natural bleach and disinfectant. Great for removing juice and food stains. Great for cleaning wooden cutting boards. I love to put lemons down my garbage disposal; with hot water, the lemon juice helps take all the gunk off the inside unit and pipes, and the rinds help pull it all down. Insects of almost all kinds (like ants) hate citrus. Rubbing lemon juice where they come in helps keep them away.

- *Club soda.* Great for getting out spots in carpets and fabric (use immediately after the spill).

- *Borax.* Great for cleaning cloths and fabric.

(See cleanser recipes in the appendix.)

## Better Choice Mom Recommends

Here are some of my favorite nontoxic cleaning products and ingredients:

- Soapworks: automatic dishwashing powder, all-purpose cleaner, nonchlorine bleach, and dishwashing liquid; Web site: www.soapworks.com

- Murphy's Oil Soap, found in any grocery store

- Top of the Mountain essential oils; Web site: www.thetopofthemountain.com

## Good, Better, Best:  **Food Preparation and Storage**

**Good:**    Keep foods away from heat sources. If you are using plastic containers, line with paper towel.

**Better:**  Transfer food into glass containers.

**Best:**    Don't buy food wrapped in plastic.

# Kitchen Pest Control

One of the most horrendous things you can do in the kitchen is to spray toxic bug killers. This is not safe or necessary anywhere in the house, but it is especially hazardous in the kitchen. The insecticide residue can be absorbed by food and remains on surfaces that food comes into contact with and on the floor where children may be crawling. The residue from professional extermination can last years inside your flooring, walls, and countertops. Beware of services that claim that they spray "safe" insecticides but require you to be out of the house during spraying. If you have to leave the house, it is toxic and definitely not safe or home friendly. Do not have spraying done.

There are ways to create a safe kitchen without toxins. The first step in ridding the kitchen of pests is to get rid of their food sources by keeping the floor clean and taking out the garbage. People buy these gigantic plastic (toxic) garbage cans that sit in the kitchen and incubate the rot inside day after day. No wonder bugs are attracted to the smell. Get a smaller stainless-steel can—one with a suction lid is best—and empty it frequently (nightly is ideal). You can also separate food waste in a smaller bag that you take out more often and use a larger bag for paper and plastic waste.

Keep dried foods like bread, muffins, and cookies in the refrigerator. If you are going to keep dried goods in your cabinets, at least keep them in glass jars so that bugs cannot smell or get into them as easily. Remember, plastic breathes, which means the bugs can smell the food. Avoid letting crumbs accumulate in cupboards. By following these steps, you can avoid bugs.

Another strategy is to find out where bugs are coming in and seal up any holes. Under the kitchen sink is often the entry point. There are holes cut out where the pipes come in, which allows bugs to crawl through under the sink and then up into drawers and cabinets. Sealing the gaps and holes around your pipes under your sink helps ensure that no bugs come in. Look for 100 percent nontoxic silicone sealants, available in most hardware stores.

Water can attract bugs, so if there is any leakage (which we also know causes mold and bacteria) in the cupboard under your sink, bugs will be attracted. To deter these bugs, you must find the leak and repair it. If neither of these measures works and bugs keep appearing, you can buy herbal mixtures to place in corners or under the sink, which will drive the critters away.

## Better Choice Mom Recommends

Cayenne pepper is an excellent way to ward off ants and flies. Sprinkle a fine line of cayenne pepper where you see bugs. If you are battling bugs, it is best not to have your kids crawling around on the floor. Bugs bring in germs from the outside. If your children do get a dose of cayenne pepper, it is nontoxic; they'll just get a little irritation on their skin or mouth. No one is going to need to call poison control; it will, however, definitely get their attention if swallowed. Lemon rinds and ground cinnamon are also useful in deterring bugs. Look for bug-deterrent recipes in the appendix.

I'm a big fan of a company called Victor Poison Free (www.victorpest .com). They have nontoxic mousetraps, ant and roach killer, and a general bug spray that works on ants, spiders, and roaches. The products work great and are safe for the home.

# Better Choice Mom Wisdom

Nothing makes me happier than to be in my own home "putzing around" in my kitchen. One of the greatest gifts that I gave my family and myself was to figure out, using a journal, what we use our kitchen for, and then to take the time to create an environment that really works for David and me.

Setting aside areas for David in the kitchen has helped him develop independence. It has also given me back a lot of my time. I had no idea how often I was being called from the other side of the house to make chocolate milk, pour juice, or fix a snack until he started doing all these things for himself. Before I reorganized the kitchen, my life was filled with "I can't find this" and "What do we have to eat?" Sound familiar?

And the organized kitchen allows it to be a *safe* kitchen. Toxic-free surfaces, safe cleansers, no dust accumulation on unused appliances, no "science experiments" growing anywhere. Now David is free to relax in his home and, better yet, thrive in the kitchen, the place where you can find him and me making a snack or hanging out talking, or David beating me at a game of chess at the counter. All these activities are so much easier for him now that he knows where to find things, has no fear of toxins in our kitchen, and isn't worrying about having a skin or respiratory reaction. The kitchen, the place of David's worst hours as an infant, is now a place for some of our best time together.

# CHAPTER 5

# The Bathroom
## Bubble, Bubble, Toxins and Trouble

What we call "Progress" is the exchange of one nuisance for another nuisance.
—Henry Havelock Ellis

THE BATHROOM has always been the place in my home where I run to wash away my troubles and temporarily escape the world. Before David was born, it was not unusual to find me soaking in the tub with candles lit and a good book in hand after a long day at work. During David's first year of challenges, the moments I could grab for myself were few and far between. Still, I managed to get in a bath and a book now and then. Nothing could clear my head better, but instead of reading a bestseller, my obsession to find out more about David's medical problems found me more often reading reference materials.

One night, just as my body began to relax and the candles to burn down, I stumbled across several reports that talked about toxins in the tub. My first thought was, You have got to be kidding! Suddenly my place of refuge was threatened. As I submerged myself in my favorite-smelling bubbles, questions began to overwhelm me.

What are in the bubbles? What are in the candles? As I moved through the reports, I began to find that not only did I need to be concerned about the bubbles and candles; I even needed to be concerned about the water.

I learned that for most of the country chlorine (see chapter 3) and other chemicals are added to our water supply. Now my nice soothing bath had become a place where my body was soaking in toxins. (For women, and especially young girls, sitting in chlorine and the other chemicals in bubble bath has been linked to several types of female problems, yeast and bladder infections being the most common, and many believe that these chemicals are causing problems with the reproductive cycle as well.) Let me tell you, I was out of the tub so quickly you would have thought I was auditioning for a horror movie.

Until this lightning bolt of information, my approach to the bathroom was how pretty I could make it. The color schemes, what mood-setting candles to use, and what would be the best lighting (or most flattering might be more honest) were my primary concerns. The truth is that these things should have been the least of my worries. The bathroom, no matter how beautiful you make it, has the potential to be the most toxic and dangerous room in your home. It is also the room in the house where much waste occurs. How many of us have dozens of products in our bathroom? Old makeup, shampoos, and an array of cleaning supplies that for one reason or another have been shoved to the back of the drawers or cabinets, collecting dust, wasting space, and, worst of all, possibly affecting your health without you even realizing it.

The government says that the amount of formaldehyde and other chemical ingredients in such products as makeup, shampoo, and body washes is not enough to be harmful, but I hope that, after reading chapter 3, common sense tells you otherwise. It did me! According to the EPA, storing under the sink one bottle of shampoo loaded with formaldehyde is safe, but who has just one of those products? What happens when three or four products that contain carcinogenic ingredients are all stored in one area? How safe is that?

At this very moment, many products in your bathroom are outgassing their chemicals into what should be a rejuvenating room in which you cleanse, beautify, and prepare to meet the world each morning or relax in a luxurious bath at night. That is why knowledge and organization, plus a whole bunch of "pitching and tossing," are key to having a bathroom that is safe, healthy, and beautiful.

## The Bathroom Journal

If you'd like to ensure your bathroom is not a toxic dumping ground, it's time to work in your journal to determine the main concerns in your bathroom, who uses it and for what purpose, and what is best for you and your family.

However you have determined to "find the purpose" of each room—whether it is by taping sticky notes on the mirror when a concern or issue arises, having family members write wish lists, or diligently writing everything down one afternoon—now is the time to begin.

Since David has his own bathroom, he was very involved in the journal process. He and I played the F.A.C.T.S. game, and boy were we amazed at what we found. From the bath mats to his toothpaste, we stripped that bathroom almost bare, and to think we thought this was a safe place! I'd already discovered that ammonia, chlorine, and formaldehyde were creeping around in my kitchen in my cleaning products and other areas, but I was not planning on these same chemicals showing up in my toothpaste, mouthwash, cosmetics, lotions, shampoo, bubble bath, and plastic toys for the tub. Between my bathroom and David's, we removed three boxes of unnecessary stuff. What had I been thinking?

Keep in mind when doing the journal that you'll probably have structural limitations, such as two basins or one, bathroom closets, a medicine cabinet, and so on. If your intention is to reconstruct the room, you'll still need to look at these elements to see what does and does not work. If the structural elements are to remain, then you'll have to work around them.

# Journal Questions: Bathroom

Whose room is this? Decide if that is the way it is to remain. For example, if you and your partner have your own bathroom but it appears that other family members are beginning to "invade," now is the time to set parameters to ensure that you get the makeover you want:

What is this room's purpose?

Are the things that are currently going on in this bathroom matching your purpose?

### Questions to help locate toxins

1. Is my throw carpet synthetic or 100 percent cotton?

2. What is my shower curtain made of—plastic or cotton?

3. Do I have wall-to-wall carpet in my bathroom? How do I clean it? What chemicals are in my spot and carpet cleaners? If I have it professionally cleaned, do I know what chemicals are being used?

4. Do I mix different products? How do those chemicals interact when mixed together in the air, and are they stored together under the sink?

5. Do I have candles in my bathroom for relaxation? Are they natural or do they have synthetic fragrances? (See appendix for candles.)

6. Do I have a convenient way to hang and dry loofa, face cloths, and hand/body towels, or am I creating a breeding ground for germs, mold, and bacteria?

7. Does my laundry basket have air flowing through to cut down on germs and bacterial growth? Do I smell the laundry basket?

8. Do I keep dirty clothes in the same closet or area as clean clothes?

9. Are my personal care products the "special of the week" instead of the healthiest products?

10. Are there gaps where the tub or shower stall meets the floor? Is there a damp or musty odor in the bathroom?

11. Are there signs of water damage or leakage in the tub or shower or under the sink?

### Questions to help organize

1. Can I get ready for my day efficiently, or do I take too long? If the latter, why?

2. Are drawers jammed with personal products, both current and from years ago?

3. How easy is it to find things?

4. How many duplicate products do I have? (Multiple duplicates may be a sign that organization is a key issue.)

5. Do I know where everything is and return each item to its proper place every time, or is one of the problems that returning the brush, mirror, or tweezers to its place is a chore?

■ ■ ■

Now the bathroom makeover begins, so roll up your sleeves, get a box or wastebasket, and start the process of eliminating what you don't use, what has expired, and what is toxic. (Make sure to dispose of toxic products correctly. You may want to have two boxes—one for easily-disposed-of items and the others for products that need to be thrown away at a proper disposal site. The latter would be any cleaners you might have or aerosol products, such as hair spray or room deodorizers.)

First, take all your products out of the cupboards and drawers and, as you go, check for an expiration date. If the item has expired, toss it. If you haven't used it in six months, out it goes. When I first went through this process, I found a can of hair spray from 1985, when the look was all about feathered hair and teased bangs. What in the world was I still doing with it in 1995?

## Beware of These Chemicals

With products you are considering keeping, check the ingredient list on the label for artificial fragrances, dyes, or toxic chemicals. Look especially for these chemicals or compounds, which are listed in *A Consumer's Dictionary of Cosmetic Ingredients* (see appendix):

*Isopropyl alcohol.* This is a solvent and denaturant (poisonous substance that changes another substance's natural qualities). Isopropyl alcohol is found in items such as hair color rinses, body rubs, hand and aftershave lotions, fragrances, and many other cosmetics. This petroleum-derived substance is also used in antifreeze and as a solvent in shellac. Inhalation or ingestion of the vapor may cause headaches, flushing, dizziness, mental depression, nausea, vomiting, narcosis, and even coma.

*Mineral oil.* This commonly used petroleum ingredient coats the skin just like plastic wrap. The skin's natural barrier is disrupted as this plastic coating inhibits its ability to breathe and absorb moisture and nutrition. The skin's ability to release toxins is impeded by this "plastic wrap," which can promote acne and premature aging. Note that most baby oils are 100 percent mineral oil. The best baby oil is made from almonds.

*Polyethylene glycol (PEG).* This is used in making cleansers to dissolve oil and grease as well as thicken products. Because of their effectiveness, PEGs are often used in caustic oven cleaners—yet they are found in many personal care products. PEGs contribute to stripping the moisture and nutrition, leaving the immune system vulnerable. They are also potentially carcinogenic.

*Propylene glycol (PG) and butylene glycol.*  As a cleaning agent or wetting agent and solvent, this ingredient is actually the active component in antifreeze. There is no difference between the PG used in industry and the PG used in personal care products. It is used in industry to break down protein and cellular structure (what the skin is made of) yet is found in most forms of makeup, hair products, lotions, aftershaves, deodorants, mouthwashes, and toothpaste. It is also used in food processing. Because of its ability to quickly penetrate the skin, the EPA requires workers to wear protective gloves, clothing, and goggles when working with this toxic substance. The material safety data sheets (the law requires all manufacturers to produce an MSDS, which lists ingredients and any precautions; see page 249) warn against skin contact, as PG has systemic consequences, such as brain, liver, and kidney abnormalities. Consumers are not protected, nor is there a warning label on products such as stick deodorants, where the concentration is greater than that in most industrial applications.

*Sodium lauryl sulfate (SLS) and sodium laureth sulfate (SLES).*  Used as detergents and surfactants, these closely related compounds are found in car wash soaps, garage floor cleaners, and engine degreasers. Yet both SLS and SLES are widely used as one of the major ingredients in cosmetics, toothpaste, hair conditioner, and about 90 percent of all shampoos and products that foam. Mark Fearer, in an article titled "Dangerous Beauty," says, "In tests, animals that were exposed to SLS experienced eye damage, along with depression, labored breathing, diarrhea, severe skin irritation and corrosion and death." The American College of Toxicology states that both SLS and SLES can cause malformation in children's eyes. Other research has indicated SLS may be damaging to the immune system, especially within the skin; skin layers may separate and become inflamed because of its protein-denaturing properties. It is possibly the most dangerous of all ingredients in personal care products. Research has shown that SLS, when combined with other chemicals, can be transformed into nitrosamines, a potent class of carcinogens that causes the body to absorb nitrates at higher levels than eating nitrate-contaminated food.

*DEA (diethanolamine) and MEA (monoethnanolamine).* DEA and MEA are usually listed on the ingredients label in conjunction with the compound being neutralized, so look for names like cocamide DEA or MEA, lauramide DEA, and so on. These are hormone-disrupting chemicals and are known to form cancer-causing nitrates and nitrosamines. They are commonly found in most personal care products that foam, including bubble baths, body washes, shampoos, soaps, and facial cleansers. On *CBS This Morning,* Roberta Baskin, one of the leading investigative consumer correspondents in network news, revealed that a recent government report shows that DEA and MEA are readily absorbed into the skin. Dr. Samuel Epstein, professor of environmental health at the University of Illinois, said, "Repeated skin applications of DEA-based detergents result in a major increase in the incidence of two cancers—liver and kidney cancers." John Bailey, who oversees the cosmetic division for the FDA, said the new study is especially important since "the risk equation changes significantly for children."

*F, D, and C color pigments.* Many color pigments cause skin sensitivity and irritation. The body absorbs most things ingested, even color. Certain dyes in some products are toxic, which can cause depletion of oxygen in the body and even death. In the eighties, one popular candy company had to ban their red candy because Red #5 was toxic. On the other hand, if you eat too many carrots, your body may take on an orangish tint, but the only negative effect is you might look a little silly. Debra Lynn Dadd says in *Home Safe Home,* "Colors that can be used in foods, drug, and cosmetics are made from coal tar. There is a great deal of controversy about their use, because animal studies have shown almost all of them to be carcinogenic."

*Fragrance.* Fragrance is present in most deodorants shampoos, sunscreens, and skin care, body care, and baby products. Many of the compounds in fragrance are carcinogenic or otherwise toxic. "Fragrance on a label can indicate the presence of up to 4,000 separate ingredients. Most or all of them are synthetic. [See chapter 3.] Symptoms reported to the FDA have included headaches, dizziness, rashes, skin discoloration, violent coughing and vomiting, and allergic skin irritation. Clinical observation by medical doctors has shown that exposure to fragrances can affect the central nervous system, causing depression, hyperactivity, irritability, inability to cope, and other behavioral changes" (from *Home Safe Home,* by Debra Lynn Dadd).

*Imidazolidinyl urea and dmdm hydantoin.* These are just two of the many preservatives that release formaldehyde (formaldehyde donors). Nearly all brands of skin, body, and hair care products, antiperspirants, and nail polish found in stores contain formaldehyde-releasing ingredients. According to the Mayo Clinic, formaldehyde can irritate the respiratory system, cause skin reactions, and trigger heart palpitations. Exposure to formaldehyde can cause joint pain, allergies, depression, headaches, chest pains, ear infections, chronic fatigue, dizziness, and loss of sleep. It can also aggravate coughs and colds and trigger asthma. Serious side effects include weakening of the immune system and cancer.

The above information is scary. My thought is forewarned is forearmed. So my suggestion is, if any of these ingredients are listed on the packaging, throw that product out!

While you're pulling out products from under the sink, look for moisture or dampness in the cabinet. If you find any, repair the problem before you put anything back in. Measure the dimensions of your drawers and cabinets to help you determine what accessories to add to help organize and define the space more efficiently. Now that the bathroom has been reduced to wide-open spaces (we hope), let the re-creating of a healthier, more efficient bathroom begin!

The next step after reducing the clutter is to address each of the main concerns that I have discovered are issues in almost every bathroom and can be troublesome for all of us if they are not kept under control. In doing this, please keep referring to your journal or notes because this is your journey and the room has to serve the needs of all who use it. Remember, you cannot get where you want to go if you do not know where the heck that is!

Here are the important issues to consider about your bathroom:

- organization
- personal care products
- bathroom cleaning products
- ventilation and air quality
- cleanliness
- cabinets and other bathroom design elements
- baths
- special concerns for children's bathrooms

## Organization

A bathroom can be a busy place! There are a lot of products found in a normal bathroom, and there are also a lot of activities that occur there. Organization is not just about the bathroom being visually pleasing; organization is key to keeping it clean, safe (toxin free), and functional.

It's hard to keep anything in its place if that place has never been defined. This is how things get shoved to the back of the cabinet and piled on top of each other, never to be found again! It is enough to drive a well-rested person crazy, let alone a tired mom who has more than a few responsibilities. So let's go back to the journal and get down to the nitty-gritty so that we can get organized.

Some common issues in the bathroom are the following:

- too many products not being used

- outdated products

- everyone's things are mixed together

- cannot find something when it is needed

- waste

To alleviate these problems, I use color coding. You'll find this tool all over my house. It is an easy way to keep things organized and an easy way to teach others what belongs where. You can use colored all-natural baskets or wire baskets or bins (which collect less dust) inside drawers to define spaces, such as yours versus someone else's, or to define categories—makeup versus hair clips and ties. I use three different-colored baskets to separate David's medicine, adult medicine, and pet medicine so that I don't have to look at the label of every bottle for an aspirin for myself. Color baskets divide hair products too—mousse and gel are separate from shampoo and conditioners.

Using the baskets has been a great way to help my son learn where his things belong, and it keeps things neat and easy to maintain. Plus you can quickly pull out a basket, look through it, and toss what is old or see what needs to be replaced. One basket can be updated in a few minutes, compared to cleaning under the sink, which can take hours—hours that I know you don't have. So by using this method of organization, you eliminate wasted space, wasted products, and wasted money. You organize once and maintain.

You can organize drawers by putting small trays (no plastic, please) in them to separate the contents. Try to keep a drawer of products that you use every day, such as makeup, hairbrush, hair clips, gel, deodorant, toothpaste, and toothbrush. Bottom drawers can be used for first aid or things that you don't use every day but to which you still want easy access.

Under the sink is usually the "yikes" area and the most troublesome for organization. Remember, if there is any moisture, do not store anything there until the problem is fixed and the area is completely dry. (Warning: As many of us learn the consequences of mold the hard way, please see my information on mold later in this chapter. It is a dangerous animal!) Again, store your items in some sort of container. If you just put things on the shelf, they get shoved to the back, pile up, multiply faster than rabbits, and are many times out of date.

As with your drawers, use separate bins for each category of item. One bin may be for hair accessories, another for personal hygiene products. A separate one can be used for first aid: bandages, corn pads, alcohol swabs, and so on. If more than one person uses the bathroom, give each person his or her own bin. If there is space in the bathroom, store each bin in its own defined space. If the bathroom is too cramped, use portable bins (such as a basket with a handle) so that everyone can bring his or her bin from the bedroom to the bathroom each morning.

## Good, Better, Best: **Organization**

**Good:**    Define a space on the countertop for personal care items so they can easily be returned to their proper place.

**Better:**    Purchase an organizer suitable for these products so they are self-contained, such as a wire bin or basket. Color coding or labeling the container is also useful.

**Best:**    Put all personal care items away and out of sight for the day, yet have them placed for easy access.

# Personal Care Products

Until my son became ill, I never thought I had a toxic product in my home. Then, after I made the connection between his illness and cleaning products, I didn't consider that the wonderful luxury items I bought for myself, such as the newest shade of lipstick, the hair product, or perfume, were harmful to him and to me. I didn't think about how often my son was on my lap, sitting on my clothes, breathing my perfume and the scent of all the other products I had splashed on, lathered up, or submerged myself in that morning. I also didn't make the connection between my "normal" everyday headaches and my choices in the first 20 minutes of every morning in the bathroom.

Now, looking back, I am shocked that I accepted headaches, feeling tired, and morning aches and pains as normal and—worst yet—feeling "just adequate" as an okay quality of life. Never for a moment did I ask why I felt lousy. I chalked it up to getting older. I could not have been more wrong.

It wasn't until I saw the agony of my child and sought answers that it began to dawn on me that chemicals might be prevalent in my home and might be harmful to a person who supposedly was not ill. I had thought that if I could just "get through the day," I was healthy. If I could "keep up" with all my responsibilities, I was being productive. Boy, was I accepting, and my new knowledge made me realize how low I had set my standards. Now, with my home free of many of the toxins that used to live with us, I can get so much more out of each day of my life, and the rewards far exceed my expectations.

Once I began to read labels, I was amazed at what they said. Where was I that I missed these warnings? Did you know that most toothpastes warn on the label that if you ingest more than a pea-size amount, you should call poison control? Poison control for something that you use in your mouth? Do you know that the manufacturers of mouthwashes warn you not to swallow their products? How can you put something in your mouth and not swallow any of it?

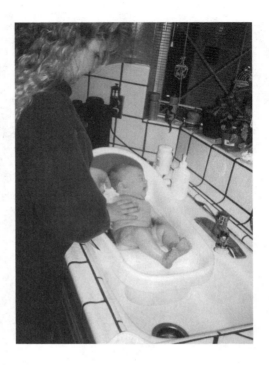

Now I know that David's "relaxing" bath was filled with liquid toxins.

How do you teach children to use toothpaste that has been colored, dyed, processed with sugar, flavored to taste like bubble gum, and filled with sparkles but to be careful not to swallow it or they may need to go to the hospital? What is up with that? If I let my son, he would eat the whole tube of bubble-gum toothpaste, and I am quite sure he would be as delighted to drink the spearmint mouthwash and the berry-berry prerinse products that have recently come on the market. When I discovered that all these seemingly harmless products were laden with chemicals that could have such devastating effects to the central nervous system and cause nausea and drowsiness, I began to see a link between David eating his toothpaste at eight months and his aggravated gums, and then his upset stomach, and cramps at two years of age. I thought I was going to scream when I discovered what these "completely harmless" products can do to sensitive adults and children.

What's more, I began to see a pattern in my journal: David's skin rash would get worse 20 minutes after I bathed him. Many times red bumps would appear all over his body, and his skin would become inflamed, scab, and then peel off in sheets. Some of these bumps were in the genital area, so his crying was definitely justified. In the beginning, I just assumed that the baby oil recommended for his cradle cap would be good all over his body and that the petroleum jelly I had always used on myself would be helpful on his red bottom. Little did I know that both of these choices were aggravating his problems. When I did research, I discovered that the baby oil and petroleum jelly are actually in a group of hydrocarbon-based chemicals refined from crude oil. (See page 250 on petroleum jelly.) And that was going on my baby's bottom? Petroleum products also attract dirt and bacteria. When our skin has to deal with this abuse every day, it is weakened, which can lead to an allergic reaction. What I was applying to my son's rashes contributed to causing the rash.

When I finally took away these toxic baby care products, I was amazed that his skin cleared up and the so-called cradle cap disappeared completely. I was so upset learning that all those painful nights were a result of my own doings. Here I was immersing him in what I thought was a soothing bath to relieve his discomfort from his rash. In reality, what I was doing was creating the rash by using bubble bath, chlorinated water, and synthetic fragrance in the bath. Added to that, I had probably scoured the tub with a toxic cleaner prior to his bath. After I took him out of the tub, I wrapped him in a towel laundered in a toxic detergent and applied some baby lotion, once again, toxic. Could I have made any more mistakes? Do you see why I was pulling my hair out? I was so easily sucked into the cute baby on the packaging, never once stopping to understand what was truly in the product.

Just as I took control of my environment, so can you—by educating yourself and then reducing your family's exposure to toxic substances. For instance, moisture and deodorant bars, which are called soap, are really a combination of bonding chemicals that act like soap. These products are now so unrecognizable to our bodies that it is a shame to even use the name "soap" in connection with them. The difference in David after bathing him with my own bar was amazing. Giving him a tubby now was a joy, not a painful chore that brought us both to tears. If you take control of the products around you, you can eliminate or prevent many health problems, including those lousy headaches and morning aches and pains! Your body is an amazing machine that will operate well unless you sabotage it by making less-than-healthy choices!

It is hard to believe, but in the process of getting ready in the morning, you may come in contact with literally *hundreds* of chemicals that are absorbed through the skin and into your bloodstream. These products include shampoo, conditioner, lotion, deodorant, hair gel, hair spray, and more. Studies show that many of these products are related to the rising increase in breast cancer among women. And we were just trying to look our best! (If you are concerned about what has been absorbed and stored in your body, there are laboratory tests that can detect the presence of these chemicals in your blood, hair, urine, fat, and tissues. See appendix, Toxin Testing.)

When evaluating your personal care products, you need to recognize that most of these products have a shelf life. After applying last year's sunscreen on one of the first hot days of the season, both David and I got a horrible sunburn. Confused as to why we got so burned despite using protection, I learned that sunscreens have a shelf life and can lose their effectiveness once the expiration date has passed. Though this may seem odd, it is best to think of sunblock as a perishable item; buying the economy size at a warehouse wholesaler is not good choice.

Keep in mind when choosing any item that the longer the item is able to last, the more preserved it is, and the more preserved it is, the more chemicals are in its formulation. Be assured, however, that you do not have to have frizzy hair or bad breath or go out of doors "sans makeup." When people first see me at public appearances, audiences are often surprised by the way I look, which is up-to-date and modern. Since I promote healthier alternatives, people expect me to look a bit more "earthy." Wrong. I love all the frou-frou that goes along with being a girl! Living a healthier life does not mean giving up luxury items or the desire to have today's "look." It just means being choosier about products. There are safer alternatives, although they do have a shorter shelf life. Do not sacrifice your health for the newest gel or latest antiaging cream.

Some may think that because these products are not mainstream (not yet anyway), they won't do the job as well as the name-brand items familiar to us from our childhood. The truth is that many of the products we grew up with can actually cause problems. An example of this is facial cleansers. You wash your face with a cleanser to remove dirt and bacteria. To remove the residue of the cleanser, you use a toner. Since the toner is actually an alcohol-based product, which dries your skin, you now apply a lotion to hydrate the skin you just depleted of its natural oils. You have just spent money (ka-ching!) on two products that the manufacturer says you must have in order to use their first product! Is this exhausting? Stop this cycle of buying more products, spending more money, and not getting the promised results. There are natural alternatives for personal care products that work. Do you think you have to use toxic underarm protection (think name-brand deodorants and antiperspirants) to smell good? Not so. Products such as the Crystal salt stone and those by Tom's of Maine work equally well and are safe. Rubbing baking soda under your arms is also a good alternative to deodorant. Better yet, eat a healthy, pure diet, and you won't need deodorant!

General product guidelines when shopping for personal care products are the following:

- Use unscented products.

- Avoid products with artificial dyes and coloring.

- Use unscented toilet paper and facial tissues.

- Avoid aluminum-containing antiperspirants.

- Avoid fluoride toothpaste.

- Products with a pump are preferable to screw-top creams or roll-ons because of bacteria growth.

- Buy things in twos so you always have a backup. You want to avoid crisis mode, when you may be tempted to buy a quick fix that would not be the best choice.

- Buy the economy-size shampoos and conditioners and refill the small container in the shower (unless there are only one or two people in your household).

Keep a permanent marker in your bathroom drawer to date your personal care products. When you buy a new item, date it right away, and throw it away if you haven't used it up in six months or by the expiration date. Set aside time once a month to go through your baskets of personal products. This has become a wonderful habit for me. Looking through my baskets, throwing or giving things away, is actually liberating! I have come to love the feeling of streamlining and simplifying life. It is only the first time that is hard!

Take five minutes at the beginning of your day and five minutes at the end of the day to give yourself a round of applause to acknowledge your hard work and the effort you are making to change. Maybe that sounds silly, but we all need positive reinforcement to recognize how far we have come and to encourage us to keep on going. I suggest you learn this "atta girl" mind-set. I promise, you will see a huge payoff in your self-esteem and confidence.

## Good, Better, Best: **Personal Care Products**

**Good:** Limit the amount of personal care products.

**Better:** Use scented products sparingly.

**Best:** Use all-natural products that are scent free or made with only 100 percent natural essential oils.

## Better Choice Mom Recommends

The following personal care products are better choices than some of the mainstream brands:

- Aubrey Organics personal care products
- Aveda personal care products
- Bio Silk hair care products
- Burt's Bees personal care and bath products
- Paul Pender's products
- Rocky Mountain sunscreen
- Salt Crystal underarm deodorant
- Soapworks bath care products
- Tom's of Maine personal care and dental care products
- Zia skin care and body products

# *Bathroom Cleaning Products*

First, define what clean is to you and what it means to the person who is sharing this room with you. Trust me—you can be worlds apart on this, and it can cause some serious problems. Who needs *that* to start the day?

When I first decided that I was going to start doing things differently in my home and get rid of chemicals, I vividly remember sitting down on my bathroom floor, opening up the cabinets under the sink, and pulling things out. Once I saw everything out of that cabinet and spread all over my floor, I couldn't get over how much stuff I had crammed into that one space. Wow!

It was very clear how many products I had that were designed to do the same chore. So why so many? Great question. As for me, I have always wrestled with products not doing what they claim to do, so I would go in search of another one that was better or offered something new. I even got sucked in by new packaging!

For cleaning the bathroom, you need something that cleans hard surfaces like counters; something that cleans your floor; something to clean your sink, tub, and shower; something to clean the toilet; something for washing your hands; and, last but not least, a window cleaner. I wanted as many dual-action products as possible and I wanted them safe for my son's health, so I created a Soapworks one that I just love. I have listed several recipes in the appendix so that you, too, can make your own cleaning products.

I know time is an issue for most of us. You can make better choices by limiting the number of products you use and store in your bathroom, so you'll clean more efficiently. Think about what chemicals are in the products you have selected and ask yourself if this is really what you want to be using.

## Hard Surface Cleaning

When cleaning a hard surface, you need to consider a few things. First, what is the surface made of? We have talked about counters and cabinets and what they are constructed of, so remember that information as you choose your cleaner. Second, what is the cleaner made of? If you are choosing a corrosive product that uses chlorine or ammonia, it will attack your counters. Third, what kind of residue will the cleaning product leave behind? That residue will come in contact with everything. One way or another, your product choice will become part of you, through hand-to-mouth contact, breathing, or touching.

## Floors

Floors are just another hard surface unless you have a special flooring material. Spot-cleaning the areas that get the dirtiest will allow you to use a gentler cleaner for all-over cleaning. Try to limit your use of heavy-duty cleaners.

## Antibacterials

I know antibacterial products are something that many of you are wild about. I have never been sold on them and don't think I ever will be. Before you decide to use these kinds of products in your home, I encourage your to do some reading. (See page 249.)

So what are in these antibacterial products? The name of the chemical is triclosan, an antibacterial agent found in products as diverse as dish soap, shampoo, toothpaste, and body washes. We first started seeing these products on the retail market in 1995. Today it's hard to find a hand soap in your grocery store aisle that doesn't contain triclosan or some other antimicrobial germ fighter.

There are two sides to every story, and that is why I encourage you to read about this chemical before just trusting that this is the choice you want for your family. From the reading and reporting I have seen on this chemical and the products that contain it, I am not at all convinced that bringing this chemical into our homes will increase our health and well-being. Most of the studies I have read (like the one conducted by the National Centers for Disease Control and Prevention [CDC] in Atlanta) say vigorous hand washing in warm water with plain soap for at least 10 seconds is sufficient in most cases, even for health care workers. So if washing the good old-fashioned way will give the same results, why add a chemical? That isn't to say that some of us may not have a need for this kind of chemical if we have a major health challenge or a compromised immune system. Just do your homework before you make this choice.

---

## Good, Better, Best: **Bathroom Cleaning Products**

**Good:**   Do not store cleaning products in your bathroom.

**Better:**   Limit the number of cleaning products. Buy ones that do more than one chore.

**Best:**   Use all-natural cleaning products, and get organized so that it takes less time to clean.

---

# *Ventilation and Air Quality*

You may think that taking a steamy shower is the cure-all for clearing up a stuffy nose, getting rid of a headache, or relaxing from the day's drama. Wrong. All that steam can cause mold, and the steam you are inhaling may contain chlorine (see chapter 3), which can trigger many health problems. Almost all municipal water has been treated with chlorine or chlorine dioxide, which can create several chlorinated pollutants, including those known as trihalomethanes ("triha what?"). One trihalomethane is chloroform, which has been linked to cancer and nervous system damage. Chloroform is released from chlorine-treated water as a vapor in hot showers.

Heavy metals, such as lead, cadmium, copper, and iron, can also be found in water from the pipes. We breathe in these pollutants as well as absorb through the skin the chlorine that has been added when we bathe or shower. The steamy water toxins can be removed with a water filter, and you can replace old, toxic pipes; however, there are more air quality issues to be aware of in your bathroom.

When I first began my search for cleaning products for the bathroom and began reading the labels on bottles, it said to use the product only in a cross-ventilated area. "Cross ventilated" means that there are windows or openings on both sides of the bathroom. I would love to see the person's house who has a window or door on each side of the bathroom. I don't have even one window in my bathroom, let alone two. So if you have cross ventilation in your bathroom, please call me, and let's have tea in your bathroom!

I do not think my bathroom is unique, yet we, the public, continue to buy these products and use them without the ventilation, without the gloves, and without the mask that the manufacturers often recommend on their material safety data sheet. Worse yet, some companies do not even mention these hazards on their labels. No wonder none of us can breathe when we come into contact with these products. Can you imagine what they do to a small child whose immune system has not matured?

Well, if we don't have cross ventilation in our bathrooms, what do we have? Exhaust systems. Unfortunately, most systems are not adequate to remove moisture or replace fresh air. Because of this, condensation from hot showers can pool, creating persistent odors, mildew, and mold. Add to that chlorine released in the air from hot showers, scented cosmetics, and aerosol hair sprays and cleaners, and the air in your bathroom can be hazardous to your well-being.

## Journal Questions: Bathroom Ventilation

### Questions about the state of bathroom ventilation:

1. Is the bathroom very damp after I shower?

2. Are towels used after showering in the morning still damp at the end of the day?

3. Does mold grow behind the toilet or under the sink? (It can appear black or green.)

4. Is there moisture in the cabinet under my sink?

5. Do I store items under a sink in a damp cabinet?

6. Is there a drip or a leak that I have ignored?

7. Are there areas where the paint is peeling or fixtures are coming loose?

■ ■ ■

If you answered "yes" to any of these questions, you need to address the ventilation and dampness in your bathroom. People often avoid dealing with moisture since it may involve having to get a plumber and tackling problems such as leaks under the sink or in the walls. Nevertheless, it is much better to get to the root of the problem than to put a bandage on it.

Do not underestimate the problems molds can cause. They have been associated with health problems such as asthma, hay fever, and arthritis. Mold is a nasty—in many cases, dire—health hazard, particularly to people with respiratory conditions such as asthma. Such individuals are especially susceptible to airborne mold, and if the problem of mold goes untreated, the individual's condition can be aggravated, and the mold will only get worse. So do not just think of mold as unsightly and a bad reflection on your cleaning ability. Think of it as a warning sign that this area of your home may be affecting how you think and feel.

## Improving Ventilation and Air Quality

To minimize the risk of breathing pollutants and to improve air quality, install shower and bath filters; their value should not be minimized or dismissed. Filters can reduce chlorine and other pollutants and can be purchased at water supply stores or on the Internet. They are fairly inexpensive. Another option is to use a crystal ball bath dechlorinator (takes the chlorine out of the water) for bathrooms where the tub faucet is separate from the shower. Make sure to replace filters regularly. If you do use oils, herbs, or salts, add them after the water has been filtered to get the most benefit out of them. What good does it do to put in a wonderful essential oil if the water is polluted?

Bathrooms should be designed so that exhaust goes outside and is not routed to an attic or garage. If your bathroom does not have a fan, install a fan in the bathroom and use the fan regularly. Even if you are one of those people who enjoy the warmth of the hot, steamy bathroom after taking a shower, at least run the fan after you are dressed so that the bathroom can air out. Open a window if you have one during or after the shower to let moisture out and fresh air in. Even leaving the door open (if privacy is not an issue) can be helpful.

Avoid aerosol hair spray, cleaners, and deodorizers. The dangers of aerosols have been well documented. Use unscented products and cleaners. Synthetic fragrances can be very toxic; potpourri can be especially irritating to a sensitive individual. Therapeutic-grade essential oils can be used for fragrance with proper instruction. Never use essential oils with direct heat, or you will lose all the benefits of the oil. (Refer to chapter 3, essential oils.) Diffusers and specially designed oil burners are much safer and are available in most health food stores. Also, avoid toxic candles. Most contain petroleum-based synthetics. Beeswax and soy candles are the safest, and, of course, unscented is best unless you purchase candles that contain therapeutic-grade essential oils. Don't use stick-on air fresheners or other devices that attach to the toilet. Eliminate the need for them by increasing ventilation, cleaning more frequently, keeping the toilet lid closed, and taking out the garbage more often. Do not spray pesticides. (See page 103 for tips on dealing with critters.)

## Good, Better, Best:  **Ventilation and Air Quality**

**Good:**     Avoid any aerosol or toxic sprays.

**Better:**  Create ventilation with a fan, open door, or open window.

**Best:**      Install a fan, ensure there are no leaks to create a mold problem, and add filters to your water so steam is not toxic.

## Better Choice Mom Recommends

### Homemade Bug Spray

In a blender, combine the following:

    1 onion
    4 cloves garlic
    2 cups water

Allow the mixture to sit overnight. The next day, strain it; put the mixture in spray bottle with water. Use this mixture as you would any other pest control. Since it is all natural, you don't need to leave the house as you do with toxic sprays.

### Commercial Anti-Pest Products/Services

Orange Mate Citrus Spray (found at Bed, Bath & Beyond, Linens 'n Things, and other major retailers)

Get Set, safe pest control, at 800-221-6188; www.getipm/sitemap.htm

Victor Poison Free Pest Control, available at home supply stores; www.victorpest.com

# *Cleanliness*

In addition to solving ventilation problems in your bathroom, there are other steps you can take to control mold and bacteria.

Most of us just have an open wastebasket. I suggest using a bathroom trash can with a lid so that the smells, germs, and bacteria are contained. Take the garbage out daily or as often as needed. Don't wait until the garbage reminds you to take it out!

Keep the lid on the toilet closed, and close it before flushing. This helps keep bacteria from spreading throughout the bathroom.

Keep the bathroom counter free of clutter (see "Organization," page 116) and wipe it daily or as needed to avoid dust and bacteria buildup. It also makes you feel better to walk into a room that is clear of distractions—less overwhelming without so much stuff!

Wash and replace bathroom towels often, and after using spread them out so they dry completely. If you have little ventilation in the bathroom, you may find that towels are still damp at the end of the day. As I said, I do not have a window, and since I live where sun is never an issue, I air my towels outside. If you don't have this luxury, you may want to fluff them in the air-only setting of your dryer.

Another area of concern when it comes to mold and bacteria is the toothbrush. Are you one of those people who avoids the dentist and gets a new toothbrush only when you are given one? Bad habit. I suggest buying a toothbrush along with products you buy on a monthly or quarterly basis. If you are Internet savvy, www.toothbrushamonth .com is an option. You automatically receive a new one in the mail every month, which reminds you to throw the old one away. All kids love to get mail, and David looks forward to receiving his personal package every month. This approach has helped me in getting him to brush his teeth as well.

Storing toothbrushes is also an issue. Many dentists recommend that you store your toothbrush in an upright position in a well-ventilated area, while others feel you should not leave it out in the open and exposed on the counter. Some put it away in a drawer, though this could be worse if it is wet. After I saw a video of what bacteria escapes into the air when the toilet is flushed and how it lands on the toothbrushes that are on the counter, I changed my habit immediately and no longer keep my toothbrush out on the counter. Whichever storage method you choose, use common sense: Rinse the toothbrush well and dry it off. You can also clean it weekly or more often with a disinfecting solution such as hydrogen peroxide or grapefruit seed extract mixed in water.

---

### Good, Better, Best:  Cleanliness

**Good:**   Get a garbage can with a lid and close the lid on the toilet.

**Better:**   Define space to limit dust and clutter.

**Best:**   Take the garbage out and dry towels every day.

---

# Cabinets and Other Bathroom Design Elements

The same issues apply in the bathroom as in the kitchen regarding cabinets (see page 83). Natural materials are preferable, such as metal and solid wood, though wood can be problematic if not treated because wood absorbs moisture, moisture creates mold, mold makes rot, and rot causes illness. So take the time to seal your wooden cabinets and other wooden furnishings with a nontoxic sealant. Cabinets can also be painted, but again, use a nontoxic paint. Avoid particleboard, which is treated with formaldehyde and other chemicals and may outgas considerably because of the heat in a bathroom.

Other sources of toxic materials in the design elements of the bathroom include flooring and walls, wallpaper, paint, carpets, and shower curtains. For more details on flooring, see chapter 4. For information on wall covering, see chapter 8, where wall treatments are covered in detail. This information can be used anywhere in your home. The key thing to remember is that if materials are toxic in one room, they are toxic in another. The bathroom can be especially dangerous because of the heat and moisture, which allows the toxics to be released at a greater speed and more often.

Ceramic tile set in a cement-based waterproof grout is the most stable and durable for floor and wall coverings. Other types of grout are treated with a silicone sealer, which is a petroleum-based product, which may not be well tolerated by some individuals. Caulk and seal all seams around tubs, showers, baseboards, and sinks to avoid moisture buildup, leakage, and mold. Plain silicone sealant may be tolerated after it is fully cured. (See Debra Lynn Dadd, *The Nontoxic Home and Office.*)

Wallpaper is absolutely not recommended. The synthetic vinyl material may be treated with phenol or formaldehyde, and the adhesives are also toxic.

Latex paints are not as durable as oil paints, and some may contain fungicides. Although they are petroleum based, oil paints are more durable, and once the solvent has evaporated and the paint has fully cured (this can be accelerated by heat and extra ventilation), oil paints are often well tolerated.

Wall-to-wall carpeting should be avoided. To say it more accurately—no way! Carpets can be extremely toxic and can be a cesspool for dust, hair, mold, and bacteria (see chapter 2). If you are not able to remove the carpet, it is helpful to dry off as much as possible or set a towel down before stepping out of the tub or shower. Bath mats and area rugs are fine if you use 100 percent cotton and not the type with the rubber or latex backing. These, too, need to be cleaned regularly, aired out, and hung to dry after using. A good reference on the hazards of carpets is *Toxic Carpet* by Glenn Beebe.

## Good, Better, Best:  **Bathroom Carpets**

**Good:** If you have synthetic carpeting in your bathroom, clean it frequently and dry off in the shower before you step out.

**Better:** Use rugs that are 100 percent natural fabric, such as cotton, and wash them frequently.

**Best:** Eliminate rugs altogether. Lay a towel down on the floor before you shower for you to step on when you get out. Then hang it up to dry afterward. Wear house slippers made from natural fabric.

Lighting is critical to the ambiance and safe use of bathroom space. It is also an opportunity for energy savings; why light the entire room when task lighting will do the trick? Choose fixtures designed for use in wet areas. In the case of recessed fixtures, insulation is critical to prevent moisture buildup.

Many bathrooms these days have an overabundance of plastics. The more you use plastics, such as shower curtains, storage containers, products bottled in plastic, towel racks, and children's toys, the more outgassing you will have. Stainless-steel, wire, and ceramic accessories are stylish alternatives.

Shower curtains can be particularly noxious. Have you ever noticed the awful smell when you open a new vinyl liner? Not a good sign. These can take a long time to outgas in a dark, closed-up bathroom; remember, heat and ventilation speed up outgassing. If you insist on using a vinyl shower curtain, fully open the curtain, place it out in the hot sun, and wait until the smell is gone before hanging it in the bathroom. Shower curtains many times are too long, so the bottom of the curtain is in water all the time. To avoid this, make sure the curtain fits the shower stall or tub. This will help reduce the problem of mold growing on the bottom. Better than a plastic shower curtain are the very pretty 100 percent cotton shower curtains you can now find. They are not only healthier but also prettier and give a different look to the bathroom. In addition, you won't have to air out a new cotton curtain before hanging it. My preference, and what I changed to, is glass doors. There are many types available, and you can even install them yourself.

## Good, Better, Best: **Shower Curtains**

**Good:** Replace your shower curtain and liner often. Look for signs of mold and make sure the curtain/liner fits properly to avoid collecting mold along the bottom edge. Stretch it out after use. Leaving it bunched up encourages mold growth.

**Better:** Use a shower curtain made of natural fabric, such as cotton instead of vinyl, and wash it frequently.

**Best:** Glass doors are preferable to shower curtains and easier to clean. Use a squeegee to clean off the glass daily. Clean the tracks of the door often with a nontoxic cleaner.

# Baths

Unless you have a whole-house water filter or a crystal ball bath dechlorinator, you should consider whether to take a bath at all. As I said earlier, I love a relaxing bath, so the investment in a water filter would have been worth it to me even if it hadn't been essential for my son, which it was. The initial investment of the filter also parlayed into additional dollars saved from fewer visits to the doctor, purchases of headache medicines, and costly trips to the spa out of necessity, not desire.

When you think of what is sitting in the bathtub, you may not be too happy about the uninvited guests. And chlorine, which is probably in your water, is being absorbed through the skin. This absorption is just as problematic, if not more so, as the chlorine in our drinking water. While each exposure may not produce a negative reaction, the cumulative effect over time can cause health problems. Many people are so desensitized to the chlorine that they do not notice the smell, but once they get a filter and the filter runs out, they can. With filtered water, you may notice a dramatic change in your skin since it will be less dehydrated without the exposure to chlorine.

Alternatives to toxic bath products are dried herbs, essential oils, and nontoxic bubble baths. (Remember that bubble baths are a no-no for little girls as they have been linked to yeast infections.) You can take fresh flower petals or dried herbs and float them on top of the water or mix them with dried milk to make a soothing milk bath. Your skin will be so soft! Dried chamomile is wonderful in a bath. It is very relaxing and a wonderful sleep aid. You can also put the herbs in plain Epsom salts, which can soothe aching muscles. Fresh or dried rosemary lifts the mood, so using this in your morning bath would be preferable. When using herbs or flowers, whether dried or fresh, make sure you use a metal strainer or cheesecloth tied with a string to prevent the drain from clogging.

You can buy bath salts that contain essential oils or make your own. If you buy your own oils, it is advisable to consult a book to guide you in the proper selection. Some companies use cheap, diluted, or synthetic oils. Only use therapeutic-grade essential oils. Be aware that "100 percent pure" does not mean therapeutic grade. (Refer to chapter 2.) Do a skin test since some oils are irritating to the skin. Dab a small amount on the inner forearm, wait 30 minutes, and then look for redness and irritation. Do not add oils directly to the water. It is best to put a little Epsom salts or sea salt in your hand, pour a few drops of the oil into the salt, mix, and then drop into the bath.

## Good, Better, Best: **Baths**

**Good:** Use all-natural essential oils in your bath.

**Better:** Use a crystal ball dechlorinator.

**Best:** Put in a water filter for the entire home.

## Better Choice Mom Recommends

Here are some products I can recommend:

- Body wash by Soapworks

- California Baby bubble baths

- Burt's Bees bath products

# *Special Concerns for Children's Bathrooms*

If you are lucky enough to have separate bathrooms for adults and children in your household, there are some special issues to consider in the children's bathroom. Here are some suggestions for their bathroom:

■ Keep cleaning products out of the children's bathroom altogether. Even if you buy fewer toxic products, kids can learn to open everything and will drink, pour out, and generally make a mess of anything they can get their hands on. Keep cleaning products in a basket or bin in a different room and transport them from room to room when you need them.

■ Trapdoor toy bins are excellent organizers (sold by www .perfectlysafe.com) for bath toys. They are made out of a rustproof wire and can be attached to the wall above the bath.

■ Install child-safe lid locks on the toilet. Keeping the lid closed cuts down on bacteria, prevents toys from going down the drain, keeps pets from using the toilet bowl as a water dish, and, most important, may save a toddler's life.

---

## Good, Better, Best: **Children's Bathrooms**

**Good:**    Keep all products away from prying hands.

**Better:**    Use all-natural products and install safety locks to limit messes.

**Best:**    Design the bathroom with children in mind to eliminate dangers. Get rid of all plastic items.

---

# *Better Choice Mom Wisdom*

It has taken time, but I have finally designed and created safe bathrooms for my son and myself. You will still find candles and soft fragrances in my bathroom; I have just made better choices in the kind I purchase. Once again, I can take a relaxing bath at the end of the day. My bathroom is free of clutter, and I can get myself together in the morning in 20 minutes, so I am able to start the day with enthusiasm instead of frustration. David's bathroom is safe for him. Gone are the plastic shower curtain and toys, toxic soaps, shampoos, and toothpaste.

As the kitchen is the heart of the home and the bedroom is the soul, the bathroom, for me, is my room for rejuvenation. Now that I have designed and organized it for me, relaxing at the end of the day is easier since I am not searching for my bath salts, loofa, robe, and incense or tripping over bath toys. Whatever you have chosen to change in your bathroom to make it healthier, enjoy the process. Embrace the changes, knowing that you are making your home a less toxic environment.

# CHAPTER 6

# The Family Room

## It's All in the Family…the Terrible Toxins Too!

Other things may change us, but we start and end with family.
—Anthony Brandt

THE FAMILY ROOM is a room that is used by the entire family (not necessarily at the same time, particularly if you have teenagers) for rest and relaxation. I remember David playing on the floor of our family room, sitting at his toy piano or rocking on his dino-rocker. While he played, I folded laundry, caught up on paperwork, or just sat and watched him. Though this appeared quite idyllic, typical for a mom and her son, there was a lot more going on in the room; who would've thought that his sitting on the couch or playing on the floor with blocks would be harmful to his health? Looking back, I recognize that the room was disorganized and that I had surrounded my son with toxic products.

One of the problems was my pigs. When I was a child, my mom gave me the nickname of "Piglet." My mother passed away when I was quite young, and one way I kept her memory alive was by collecting pigs. Each had a special meaning, and I loved each one dearly. I never thought there would be a day when I wouldn't have my pigs.

But David's multiple chemical sensitivities forced me to reevaluate my choices in my home, and I came to see my pig collection for what it really was: a dust collector, a distraction, and a money pit. My pigs were a cozy place for dust, dust mites, and germs to land on and accumulate, and the five or ten dollars I spent a week on a new pig was in direct conflict with what I needed to be doing, which was creating a safe home for David. The less clean and clear space you have, the harder it is to build a safe home.

When I first decided to get rid of my pig collection, I couldn't do it because there was a great deal of emotional attachment. To help me "ease into it," I began by getting rid of other things that were easy to let go of. By the time I came to my collection of over 200 pigs (I know, I know—that is a lot!), I was ready. I let everybody know that I was letting the pigs "out of the barn" and that they could take any that they wanted. I donated some to thrift stores and literally dumped the rest. I kept two—one from my dad and one from David. Now every time I see a pig, I just smile.

After streamlining my home room by room, I can clean more quickly, and I'm more focused on what we want to accomplish in a day. And yes, dumping the pig habit also helped me realize that I was spending money on a needless item that gave me a short "feel-good high" that had no purpose. To help me break the habit, I began putting the money that I would spend on another pig into a jar. What a great party I had the following year, funded by my "piggy" bank!

The problems that need to be resolved in the family room are how to make healthy choices with regard to hidden toxins and how to design the room so that it functions effectively for each member of your family. Sitting on the floor is fine unless you are sitting on carpeting. Watching television can be relaxing unless you are sitting on a couch that has been treated with a fabric protector or you have to

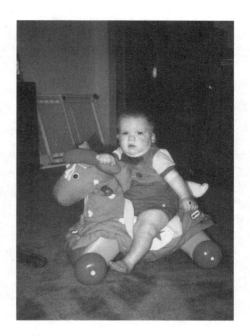

The dino-rocker was David's beloved friend. Unfortunately, his "friend" was filled with chemicals. An added whammy—I washed Dino's removable head in detergent, and David often chewed on his mane. If riding wasn't bad enough!

sit three feet away from the television screen (and its accompanying electromagnetic fields [EMFs]) because the room is "overstocked."

Since the family room is where you gather and in some cases entertain, it should be warm and inviting. You need to decide if you want it to be a showplace or are more interested in creating an intimate atmosphere with simple furnishings. This room is a great place to express your personality, yet at the same time you need to make sure that what is in the room—flooring, bookcases, electronics—is not defeating the purpose of rest and relaxation or triggering allergic reactions or other unpleasant symptoms. When you're thinking about remaking your family room, consider these important areas: storage, the right type of furniture, flooring, lighting, and wall and window coverings.

Many times our homes evolve according to changing needs, and we just add or accommodate without thinking things through and taking the time to reorganize. As with the kitchen and bathroom, you need to become a detective in order to make necessary changes. Notice how your mood, attitude, and energy level change after spending a while in the family room. This will provide clues to things you may not have realized. Maybe you get a headache when you read in this room because there is not adequate light. Maybe you get the sniffles because the couch and the many overstuffed pillows are loaded with dust mites or sprayed with Scotchgard. Journaling can help you follow the clues and reveal the real nature of any health problems associated with this room.

## The Family Room Journal

You can start the family room journal by considering what the function of the family room is and how you would like everyone to participate in this room. The room needs to be designed to accommodate all the family members who use it and all the activities that go on there. This means that if there is one television and a video game system is hooked up to it, only one of these two activities can be happening at a time (and generally what happens is conflict!). Loud toys in this room may interfere with someone watching television or reading or with others playing a game.

If there is clutter or overcrowding, you want to survey the room to see if there are objects that really do not belong or do not have a designated space. Just as important, is this really the best place for some of these activities? Can children really do their homework when the television is on? Is this a habit you want to cultivate? Is the computer in a good location with proper lighting? What about the chair that you use for the computer? Is it there because it matches the decor of the room, or is it really the right type of chair for working at a computer?

Do you have too many knickknacks in this room? This room should express your personality, but sometimes we get carried away. Have you been to one too many craft fairs? Have your collectibles begun to take over your "practicables"? What may look cute by itself becomes, in excess, a visual nightmare and a dust depository. Start a new rule: You cannot add anything unless you get rid of something. Before you buy anything new for the room, consider it as something that you have to dust. Do you really want to add to your workload? Perhaps consider quality versus quantity.

If each family member brings something to the family room to work on and then leaves it there, pretty soon you have total chaos. Laundry, sewing, newspapers, puzzles, toys, and homework are some of the many things you often see strewn around a family room. What should be a relaxing place can become an obstacle course.

Change your family's bad habits or accommodate. If the kids always drag their favorite toys from their bedrooms and leave them in the family room, why fight it? Just create a basket or area for the toys they use in this room. They may be more likely to put them away if there is a place right there, just for them. If you sew in the family room, buy a little shelf or cabinet just for sewing items so that they will be contained in a specific place. If you have a computer in the family room, make sure you have enough shelves or space for all the accessories you need, such as paper, disks, and computer books. When at all possible, put the basket of toys in a closet out of sight. By doing this, you are less visually bombarded with "stuff" as you enter the room.

# Journal Questions: Family Room

### Questions to help locate toxins

1. Do the furnishings add to health problems? Is there plastic on the couch, Scotchgard on fabric furniture, or pillows that have not been cleaned?

2. How do I feel when I enter the family room? How do other family members feel when they enter this room?

3. Are there candles in the room that might have synthetic fragrance?

4. How many electronics are plugged in, and are they all necessary?

5. Do pets have a place to sleep, or do they use the same furniture we use?

6. Do we eat in this room? If so, are spills and crumbs cleaned up so bugs and mildew won't be a problem?

7. What type of flooring, cabinets, and window coverings do you have? Do these add to the "toxic overload"?

### Questions to help organize

1. What is the function of this room?

2. How would I like everyone to participate in the family room?

3. Do all family members who use this room feel that they have their own defined space?

4. Is there clutter or overcrowding?

5. Are there objects that really do not belong here or do not have a designated space?

6. Is this really the best place for some of the activities that go on in this room?

7. If there is a computer, is it in a good location with proper lighting?

8. Is there adequate seating for everyone?

■ ■ ■

The family room is going to require a group discussion since everyone spends time in this room. Family dynamics can get played out or revealed in this room. Is there one person in the family who leaves things lying around and whom you always have to nag to pick up after themselves? Does this create tension, which leads to arguments? Or does mom just pick up after everyone else and resent it? These dynamics are common.

A few years ago I alleviated this whole drama for myself. If I find something where it does not belong, I throw it out. After warning David about my new policy over a few days, I found his favorite shoes once again where they were not supposed to be, so they were donated to charity. This cost me $29.99, but he learned very quickly to put his things back where they belong. This approach to organization has taught him to be on my team and not create more work for us.

The following are the main issues in the family room:

- flooring
- lighting
- furniture
- window treatments and wall coverings
- electromagnetic radiation from entertainment equipment
- ventilation and air quality
- cleaning products
- children's area

## Flooring

People often think of the family room as a cozy, homey place to snuggle up and watch movies or television. For many, a hardwood or tile floor does not fit into this picture. You may think you need wall-to-wall carpeting so people can sit on the floor. I mentioned that the first place to change flooring is the bedrooms. I would say this room is probably second in importance because children and adults often sit or lie on the floor in this room.

I really encourage you to let go of the idea of carpeting in the family room. Breathing outgassing formaldehyde, dust, and mold is not conducive to relaxation. Put in safe flooring and find other ways to make the room cozy, such as with nontoxic area rugs, floor mats, or big pillows. It also makes sense to have a more durable floor surface such as hardwood because there is usually more traffic in this room than in other areas of the house. It may take time to get used to, but the positive health benefits are worth it.

A good idea is to buy a mat where your children and their friends can play. This defines a specific area just for them. You can use a yoga mat or gym mat. There are mats made of less toxic materials than vinyl, such as 100 percent organic cotton; you can get these from the same distributors that sell safe bedding. The benefit of using a mat is that you can roll it up and place it behind or under a couch when not in use, and you can wipe it off when it gets dirty. Some have covers that you can remove and throw in the wash.

## Good, Better, Best:  **Flooring**

**Good:**    If you keep carpeting, put something between you and the carpeting if lying on the floor, playing games, and so on.

**Better:**    Use nontoxic cleaners.

**Best:**    No wall-to-wall carpeting. Install all-natural, durable flooring.

## Better Choice Mom Recommends

The following are sources for children's play mats:

www.ayurvedahc.com

www.greenmarketplace.com

www.yogamats.com

# *Lighting*

Lighting design for the family room needs to take into consideration all the different activities that go on in the room. Some guidelines to use for lighting are as follows:

- general lighting for entertaining and watching television
- task lighting for reading, sewing, or children's play or homework
- accent lighting for painting, art, or plants

Dimming controls for overhead lights and torchière lights are becoming popular and are ideal in the family room to adjust for different moods. Lamps should be used for task lighting, while mini–track lights or portable cans can be used to accent artwork and plants.

Do not use halogen bulbs. They are a fire hazard, get very hot, and use five times the electricity of a standard lightbulb. If you like the look of a lamp, generally you can buy that design with a regular bulb attachment, and then you can use a full-spectrum bulb. Remember to avoid fluorescent light; replace with full-spectrum bulbs whenever possible, especially for task lighting. This reduces electromagnetic radiation and more closely simulates natural sunlight (refer to chapter 2).

## Good, Better, Best: **Lighting**

**Good:** Consider what is being done in the room and make sure there is adequate lighting for each of those activities.

**Better:** Turn on lights only when needed for those activities to eliminate volatile organic compounds (VOCs).

**Best:** Do not use halogen bulbs. Use full-spectrum lighting.

# *Furniture*

There is no way around it—environmentally safe furniture is more expensive than its toxic counterpart. You have to pay more for real wood (no particleboard) and all-natural fabrics and fillers that are untreated (organic). Adding unsafe furnishings to a house, however, can triple the inhabitants' chemical exposure, leading to health problems, which means potentially more trips to the doctor—and there is nothing inexpensive about that! Also, if you invest in a good-quality couch, it will last much longer.

So what do you do? The best choice is to realize the importance of health and make your decision on that basis. We always somehow find the money for things we really want. Women will gripe in the grocery store that organic fruit is 50 cents more per pound than the same fruit grown conventionally, yet they think nothing of spending $200 on moisturizers and antiaging creams. The irony is that the organic fruit is going to have more of an effect on what your face looks like in 10 years than the makeup will.

If you are chemically sensitive, then you have to pay extra for nontoxic furnishings. If you are not, then you can decide how much you want to invest.

Just as chemicals on clothing, bedding, and mattresses can compromise our health, so too can those on couches. Companies cannot afford to have mold and bacteria accumulate during shipping, so products are bombarded with all sorts of chemical treatments. (And, truth be told, many consumers like the "protection" against spills offered by such sealants.) Scotchgard is the one most familiar to us. You know how we all had a relative with a plastic-covered couch when we were growing up? Well, the plastic covering is still on some sofas sold today; the only difference is its form: Scotchgard and sealants are all derived from plastic. We just can't see it!

Again, unless you specifically search out fabrics and fillers that are 100 percent organic, untreated cotton, you can assume the products have been treated. Even products labeled organic may have been treated. Beware of companies that use organic cotton but say they have to wrap the products in wool to comply with federal flammability standards. You have to ask specifically if the products were treated with flame retardants. Always ask questions. Do not wait until you get a product home to find out that a member of your family cannot tolerate it well.

Besides preventing mold growth, why do we have chemicals such as Scotchgard on couches and sealants on carpets? The answer is generally so we can more easily clean up spills. Why do we have spills? Because people are eating all over the house instead of in a defined area. This makes messes and stains, invites bugs, and grows bacteria. Why not save yourself the grief and confine eating to only certain areas of the house? Why poison ourselves every day breathing toxic chemicals so that we can be prepared for the messy spills we could have avoided in the first place? If you are going to eat in the family room, get stacking tables that fold up and can be put away after you have completed your meal. Breakfast serving trays with little legs that you can put on the floor are also suitable. Create some boundary or some containment for the food and mess and leave the Scotchgard behind.

## Options for Couches

Most family rooms have a couch. It's the biggest piece of furniture in the room and probably the most used. Since David and I spent so much time on the couch, from breast feeding to story time to now playing card games, I put a lot of thought and money into making this purchase be the absolute best possible one for us. I bought a huge couch, one with big pillows that comfortably accommodates both of us. The fabric is all natural and has not been treated, and the pillow covers can be removed, shaken, and aired out. If you are not able to replace your couch, at least consider new nontoxic covering for the cushions. Leather, which is well tolerated by many, creates a barrier from dust mites. The downside is that most solutions used to treat the leather are highly toxic. Though it can be expensive, I use mink oil to treat our leather couch in the formal family room. You may have to experiment with different products to find what works for you.

One hundred percent organic cotton couches are great but expensive, and patterns and styles of fabric are limited (however, manufacturers are finally listening to the consumer, so there are certainly getting to be more choices). A futon made of 100 percent organic cotton is less expensive than a traditional couch, can work as a bed, and is environmentally safe, but some feel that they are not very comfortable for sitting or sleeping on. One benefit to futons is that you can purchase different coverings. So if you're a bit neurotic (and I mean that in the nicest way) and get bored easily with the same look, a futon might be your best choice.

If you're not able to replace the couch, you can give the room an ozone treatment to break down and eliminate chemical odors and outgassing fumes. Or try an air filter in the room.

## Good, Better, Best: **Furniture**

**Good:** If you cannot change the furniture or filling, treat it with ozone to break down and eliminate chemical odor or take it outside to air. Place an air purifier in the room.

**Better:** If you can't replace the couch, replace the fabric or filling since it was most likely treated with Scotchgard or other chemicals.

**Best:** Buy furniture frames of untreated wood or metal. Buy fillings and fabric that are 100 percent organic, untreated cotton or another natural material, such as leather.

## Better Choice Mom Recommends

The following are sources for environmentally safe furniture:

- Bright Future Futon: 505-268-9738

- Pure Seasons: www.pureseasons.com; 800-721-3909; P.O. Box 1206, Sausalito, CA 94966

- Real Goods Trading: www.realgoods.com
- Green Babies Organic: www.greenbabies.com
- SimplyNaturalHome: www.simplynaturalhome.com
- Tiny Tush: www.tinytush.com

## Window Treatments and Wall Coverings

The priorities with window treatments are that they be something that can be taken down and washed, by hand or machine, and that they be made from 100 percent organic untreated cotton if at all possible. Wood blinds or shutters are an option as long as they are not treated with toxic chemicals. Don't buy plastic, such as in miniblinds, which collect dust and are hard to clean, which means most people don't keep up with cleaning them.

Do not dry-clean curtains, or you will be introducing formaldehyde, perchloroethylene, and other toxic chemicals to outgas in a room that is supposed to be relaxing. If you insist on taking curtains to the cleaner, ask for steam cleaning or more ecologically safe cleaning, such as "wash and fold," so that they don't use chemicals for cleaning. If you dry-clean your window coverings, at least hang the curtains outside to air until you no longer can smell the chemicals before you bring them into the house again. Also, bring the curtains home from the cleaners in the car trunk, not in the passenger part of the car. You will get a heavy dose of toxins just by driving with them hanging in the backseat, especially if you don't come home right away but run errands and leave the curtains sealed in the hot car each time you get out. You may think you are tired, cranky, and headachy because you have been running around all day, but maybe it is because you have been incubating in chemicals. Be suspect if you or others have a Dr. Jekyll/Mr. Hyde kind of personality change when you have been inhaling toxins such as these. Before I stopped buying clothes that needed to be dry-cleaned, I thought I was being so careful by airing the clothes out before they went into my closet. It didn't cross my mind that David was in his baby seat right next to the dry cleaning on the way home. These things are simple, but habits are hard to break.

Again, I love simplicity. Less is better. I like the sun and an open-air feeling, so I do not want dark, heavy toxic curtains that have to be dry-cleaned. Who says you have to have anything on the windows at all? Many people think they are making a fashion statement with curtains. Try showing your good taste and flair for interior design in other ways.

As for wall coverings, the same concepts I've already discussed apply to the walls in the family room. Wallpaper is not a good choice. Avoid toxic paints; use paints with lower VOCs. Another thing to consider for this room is hanging tapestries, oriental rugs, or nice prints to liven up the room. While these may not be totally chemical free, they are a better choice than layers of toxic paint or wallpaper. See chapter 2 for details about wall coverings and paint options.

## Good, Better, Best: **Window Treatments and Wall Coverings**

**Good:** If you have to keep the curtains you have and dry-clean them, let them air outside for several days before returning them to the house.

**Better:** Keep what you have but do not dry-clean. The alternative to dry cleaning is steam cleaning or using cleaners who use "green" cleaning agents.

**Best:** Buy 100 percent organic, untreated curtains that you wash at home or wood shutters or blinds.

# Electromagnetic Radiation from Entertainment Equipment

Electrical outlets and electrical cords are much like a water pipe. The pipe always has water in it, not only when you turn on the faucet. Your electrical cords and outlets always have electricity in them, and a flip of the switch activates it. This does not mean you are not getting EMFs if the switch is off. You are. That's why I encourage you to evaluate how many electronics are in the room and if the cords and outlets are really necessary. For a refresher on EMFs, see chapter 2.

Entertainment centers can get crowded with many electronics, which add a source of electromagnetic radiation to your family room. Plug your electronic equipment into a power strip so that you can turn it all completely off at night or when not in use.

You can also have the entertainment center connected to a light switch on the wall, which can be easier to reach than a power strip on the floor behind the unit. Also consider if you really use everything you have plugged in. If you have a DVD player and rent most of your movies in that format, do you really need the VCR? How many of us have the lamp on while watching television, and for what reason?

To avoid EMFs, make sure that no one sits too close to the television or other electronic equipment and that the children's play area is not right near the entertainment center. Six feet away from the television screen is a general guideline for distance; larger televisions have a larger field of exposure, so safe distances can vary. Plants placed on top of or on the shelves of an entertainment center can be visually appealing and help counteract radiation. Certain stones and crystals can also combat electromagnetic pollution. For more detailed information on the healing power of crystals, see *Love Is in the Earth,* by Melody R. R. Jackson.

## Good, Better, Best:  Electromagnetic Radiation from Entertainment Equipment

**Good:** Unplug electronics when not in use.

**Better:** Use green plants in the room to help counteract radiation.

**Best:** Limit the number of electronics in the room and put in a switch to stop power.

# *Ventilation and Air Quality*

The issues of air quality can be more complicated in the family room than in smaller rooms such as bedrooms. This is because the family room is larger, often has no doors, is connected to other rooms such as the kitchen, has more furnishings that may be outgassing, and has a heavy traffic flow.

In small rooms, air filters can be effective in reducing airborne contaminants, but the door and windows have to be closed and the room contained for the unit to be effective. In the family room, filtration may be less effective since there may not be doors sealing this room. You definitely need a larger air purifier. Most air purifiers filter particulates and do not contain media that effectively reduce VOCs or formaldehyde in the air. You have to research and find units that specifically have activated charcoal or other media that absorb chemicals.

Bringing in an air purifier needs to be combined with reducing the output of chemicals into the family room's air. It does not make sense to put an air purifier next to new furniture that is outgassing formaldehyde. The filters in the purifier will get saturated right away and will then be ineffective. You have to do both: reduce the chemical output by getting rid of outgassing material and filter the air.

Many family rooms have several windows, so cross ventilation can be a good way to air out the room, though this won't work if you live in a highly polluted area.

## Good, Better, Best: **Ventilation and Air Quality**

**Good:** Eliminate toxic furnishings in the family room.

**Better:** Open the windows regularly to circulate the air.

**Best:** Buy a large room air purifier for the family room.

# Cleaning Products

Since your family room gets used a lot, it probably gets dirtier than some other rooms in the house. If you take the time to make the furnishings as toxin free as possible, don't use cleaning supplies that reintroduce the toxins and chemicals into the space!

## Carpet and Furniture Stain Removers

You must be a savvy shopper when buying cleaning products. Many products claim to be natural, safe, or nontoxic and to clean miraculously—spots, stains, and all! But beware of trickery and good marketing. For example, one popular stain remover claims this: proven safe, nonirritating, no hazardous chemicals, does not deplete the ozone, and biodegradable. But the label (you're reading them regularly, right?) reads this way: harmful if swallowed; may be fatal; wear gloves while using this product; and avoid prolonged skin or fingertip exposure. Does this sound like a safe, nontoxic product to you? Do you want to risk your health just to get a stain out? You do not even want a product like this in your house, especially if you have children. Companies are not being policed to make sure they adhere to marketing claims, so you have to take responsibility to examine the products you use, see if they make sense, and choose wisely. No government agency or company is going to protect our health or the health of our children. That is the power we have as moms. By not buying these products, we are protecting our family and telling the manufacturers we don't want products that poison.

Manufacturers of cleaning products are not required to list ingredients on the label, so it is important that you take on the responsibility of investigating the products further to see if they are safe. If you do not have time to read labels, familiarize yourself with safer product lines, health food stores, or on-line distributors of safer products. If you are unsure whether a product is unsafe, the warnings themselves can alert you. Remember, a label that says "caution" is a less toxic product, such as an eye irritant, but not at all life threatening; "warning" requires further investigation to find out what the warning is; and "danger" indicates a more toxic product and is a no-no in my world.

Having carpets professionally cleaned is not advised because they use chemicals you do not want in your house. It is better to have a great vacuum cleaner and simply clean stains with an all-purpose or carpet cleaner immediately after spills. If you have to have the carpet shampooed, rent a machine yourself and use your own nontoxic cleaner (see appendix under recipes). Make sure to rinse out the machine first to remove the residue of previously used chemicals. All this hassle is even more reason to have hardwood, tile, or marble floors.

## Dusting Sprays

Products used for dusting, which you spray on wood, coffee tables, furniture, or bookcases, are absolutely hideous; they can be filled with as many as 5 to 10 chemicals, all in the name of removing dust. Instead of launching into a long discourse on the many toxic ingredients that we have repeatedly discussed, I'll ask you to simply consider this: These dusting sprays are not necessary to get things clean. The purpose or definition of dusting is to collect and remove dust from the environment. You do not need an oily, gooey, smelly spray to accomplish this. These products do not enhance your cleaning, and they endanger your health with the buildup of toxic residue on the furniture.

Dust with a wet rag or use your vacuum cleaner. Afterward, you can simply apply a small amount of oil, such as olive oil, to wood furniture to moisturize it and make it shine. If the furniture is not real wood, then it does not need to be treated at all. I am a big fan of the "One Cloths," "Mystic Maid Cleaning Wipe," and microfiber cleaning cloths now available at your grocery or home supplies store. (Take note, however, that some microfiber cleaning cloths now contain chemicals, so buy from a "safe" company.) These microfiber cloths make dusting a breeze and also work great on stainless steel. (My refrigerator has never looked as great as it does since I've been using these types of cloths.) You can wash the microfiber cloths and reuse them forever—a good investment.

## Aerosol Room Fresheners

You freshen indoor air by opening a window or running an air purifier—period. Aerosol products that claim to clean the air and reduce the amount of bacteria are extremely toxic. The common brand-name ones contain hydrochloric acid, formaldehyde, and isopropyl alcohol. Hydrochloric acid is so caustic that it can burn the skin and respiratory tract. You may kill a few microscopic bugs with one of these sprays, but you also introduce a carcinogen, a respiratory irritant, and a skin irritant. These sprays can induce an asthma attack in some people. Go to the source of the problem; don't create a worse one.

If the air ducts in your house are really dirty with mold and bacteria, it does not make sense to spray a toxic chemical to kill bacteria in the air. Clean the ducts, and then the air will be better (see chapter 2). Good cleaning habits, vacuuming and dusting, and using fresh flowers, dried herbs, or essentials oils can make a room smell fresh—naturally.

---

## Good, Better, Best:  **Cleaning Products**

**Good:**    Eliminate toxic cleaners as much as possible.

**Better:**   Buy all-natural cleaners. Use oils for polishing.

**Best:**    Limit the number of dustables and conquer the source of toxins with an air purifier.

---

# *Children's Area*

The place where your children play can be a real breeding ground for germs, bacteria, dust, and pests such as ants. Since a child's immune system is much more sensitive than an adult's, you really need to examine what is in this area as well as keep it clean.

## Play or Activities

Baskets for certain toys and activities are an excellent way to organize children's playthings in the family room, plus they make it easier for the children to take out and put away their things. To simplify life even more for them, create different baskets for different toys suitable for that room. For example, I would not allow play dough, Silly Putty, or messy toys in the living room, but they are fine for the kitchen because it is easier to clean up there. The family room basket has quiet toys, such as Etch-a-Sketch, that the kids can use while others are watching television or reading. Louder toys go in the bedroom (please!). This way, children know which toys can be played with in each area.

Things flow smoothly when everyone can have input, their needs are considered, and there is logic in the way things are arranged.

## Homework or Relaxation

In *Is This Your Child?* Doris Rapp, M.D., documents cases of children whose handwriting was affected by their exposure to allergens or chemicals. This indicates that our noses, skin, and lungs are not the only body parts affected by allergies; our brain can also be affected. Children's ability to think, learn, and perform well in school can be negatively influenced not only by the environment at school but also by the one at home. If your children have difficulty concentrating or doing homework, there may be something irritating in the area where they are trying to study. It could be a particleboard desk, toxic paint, toxic carpet, or electronics emitting electrical pollution. Changing the area where they do their work could help them concentrate. I advise making a "safe" room, such as the bedroom, and have that be where they study and do homework.

You also need to consider whether homework can get done if others are talking or watching a video or television. If your child wants to be "part of the family" while doing homework, make sure that the assignment is completed in a legitimate amount of time and that the distractions are not affecting the quality of work. Also make sure that the area is set up to do homework, with good lighting, a chair, and a desk. If this is not what you have defined for this room, then homework needs to be done in the right environment. Until this year, David had always done his homework in his bedroom.

Now I find that he doesn't want to do it in his room; rather, he wants to do it where I am. Because many nights I work in my office, I have now set up an area where he can bring his schoolwork and be with me. Perhaps because I have been gone so much lately, he needs more "mommy time." This is just another example of the fact that your life continues to evolve and that creating a healthier home is not a one-time event but changes all the time, depending on the dynamics of what is happening in your home.

## Good, Better, Best: **Children's Areas**

**Good:**  If you allow your children to do homework in the family room while other family members are watching television or doing other activities, set a timer and be aware of how long it takes them to complete assignments.

**Better:**  Children do homework in the family room with no television or activities going on to distract them.

**Best:**  Children do homework at a desk in a separate room with no distractions, good lighting, and no outgassing furnishings.

# Better Choice Mom Wisdom

It can be overwhelming and frustrating to learn how saturated and bombarded we are by chemicals every day. It may feel like a huge job to get them out of your life, and you may find yourself thinking, "Why bother?" When I first started, I wondered—and still wonder at times—whether all this work was really worth it. I "fall off the wagon" and drink a Diet Coke or take some clothing to the dry cleaners because, no doubt about it, sometimes it's quicker and easier. Then I feel awful. I know this inner struggle between health and convenience is good for me because each time I fall back into my old habits, I come back even more committed to making better choices.

Again, decide which changes you want to implement first in the family room and involve your team. Do *not* take on too many things at once. Make a plan to implement small changes slowly, over time. If you try to take on everything at once, it will feel like too much, too soon, and too fast, and you will want to give up no matter how determined you think you are right now. Take things in stages. Certain things, such as pulling up carpet, replacing furniture, or purchasing air purifiers, will take a significant amount of time, thought, and money. Other changes you can implement right away, such as replacing toxic cleaners with safer ones and reorganizing your space. Remember, the purpose of all this is a safer, healthier, better future for you and your family.

# CHAPTER 7

# The Living Room and Dining Room

## Overstuffed, Overdecorated, Overdone

Destiny is not a matter of chance, it is a matter of choice; it is not a thing to be waited for, it is a thing to be achieved.
—William Jennings Bryan

TO THIS DAY, the concept of a formal room makes me say, "Give me one good reason!" I know for many of you this room has been decorated with painstaking attention to every detail. My mom had a beautiful living room for company that my brother and I called the "blue room" because of the wall-to-wall blue carpeting. It also had a floor-to-ceiling mirrored wall on one side of the room, which magnified all that we did; a cabinet-style Magnavox hi-fi stereo hung with curtains to hide the speakers; and a big, heavy *Gone with the Wind* type of curtain on the other side of the room.

We used to sneak into the room, turn on the stereo, and watch ourselves dance in the mirrors. With the light coming in from the windows, we would see sparkles in the air. It was like magic. Unfortunately, we were easily caught because my mother raked the carpet each week so that all the carpet pile was neatly going the same way.

The "dancing footprints" we left behind were a dead giveaway that we had invaded this space. I can probably count how many times this room was actually used for company. I also now know that the beautiful sparkles we danced in were dust in the air because who thinks you need to dust a room that is never used?

In this book, I cover the living and dining rooms together because these two rooms are often used when entertaining. They may have more expensive furnishings than other rooms in the house because people may want to showcase their best things. These generally are also the rooms that many kids are told are "off limits." Mom does not want anyone playing in there where fine china can get broken or stains can end up on an expensive couch. I have a very different perspective now that I completely overhauled my house to make it healthier. That was an enormous expense, so why not spend the most money where you spend the most time? Therefore, I initially did not focus my attention on these two rooms since they are used less frequently. These rooms are where I allow the most "mistakes" in terms of being health friendly. I did not spend a lot of money changing the flooring or furnishings in the living and dining areas until I had created a safe bedroom, kitchen, and family room. That doesn't mean I don't thoroughly cover the issues of these rooms in this chapter. I guess what I am saying is to keep an open mind when approaching this area of the house. When you write in your journal, really examine how the room is used and what you need to do to ensure your family's health.

## The Living and Dining Rooms Journal

Keep in mind the question, Do you really need a stuffy, overblown showcase filled with doo-dads? The first thing to explore in your journal is how often the living and dining rooms are really used. For some people, holidays are the only time they are in these rooms, while others may have Sunday dinner there every week. If you use this area only

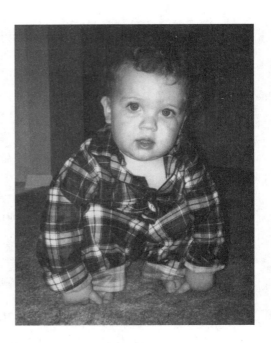

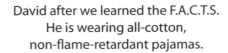
David after we learned the F.A.C.T.S.
He is wearing all-cotton,
non-flame-retardant pajamas.

once or twice a year, does it really make sense to spend a lot of money on expensive furnishings? The reality for me is that my company always ends up in the kitchen anyway. If you do not use the living/dining area as it is set up, think about changing it. Yes, throw away tradition! Be daring! Be unconventional! Do what works for you. After all, that mortgage you are paying ought to give you some rights!

When I began working on this room, I took the couch and frou-frou furnishings out of the living room and moved in a pool table, stereo, dartboard, and pinball machine and now have a room that is used all the time. It also sent a message to my son that I would rather have him play a game than sit in front of the television. Even better, since we are the only family on the block with a game room, David and his friends spend a lot of time at my house. Since I travel so much, it is a real gift to be able to maximize my time with my son, listen to the chatter of him and his friends, and remember how I once thought I was just as superhuman as they believe they are.

I then took the dining room and converted it into my office. One of the life decisions I made after David got sick was that I was not going to commute to my son anymore. Having an office at home rid me of working in a cubicle (don't rats do that?), plus it allowed me to take part in David's life even more by seeing the smiles (and tears), the unexpected discoveries, and all the wonders that happen to a child.

# Journal Questions: Living and Dining Rooms

### Questions to help locate toxins

1. Are there any decorations that might be toxic that I can remove? This includes toxic candles, curtains, tablecloths, or other synthetic materials.

2. Are there too many decorative items?

3. Do I keep up with the dusting and generally maintain this room?

4. Does each item in the room add to the quality of the environment or take away from what I am trying to create?

### Questions to help organize

1. Is this room overflowing with things that have nowhere else to go (papers, books, or other things)?

2. How often do I use the room?

3. Why isn't it used more?

4. Is there a real need for the room as it is designed, or could I maximize the function of my home by using this room for another purpose?

5. Is this an adults-only room? Is that what I want it to be?

6. Is this room a relaxing or inviting environment for guests, or has it become stuffy and formal?

■  ■  ■

If a game room or an office does not suit your needs, perhaps consider a specialty room for your hobbies, a television/video game room, or even a room where your family can go for quiet time without any stimulation. For many of you, this may not be what you want, but my point is that unless "your space runneth over," use the space wisely and make a room that you will use and enjoy. If you choose to keep the dining and living rooms, getting feedback from the rest of the family with a team approach is still a good idea, even though most often I find that these areas are mom's domain.

The following are issues of concern in the living and dining rooms:

- flooring

- ventilation and air quality

- furnishings

- decorating

## Flooring

In most houses, the living and dining rooms have wall-to-wall carpeting. You know by now how I feel about that! Plus, carpeting in the dining area is really a bad choice. Food spills are inevitable and are nothing more than a hassle to clean, and if the carpet is not maintained, food spills can encourage mold and bacteria growth.

We have discussed in previous chapters the ideal flooring—marble, ceramic tile, hardwood—but at first glance, it may seem cost prohibitive. However, if you evaluate the long-term cost, including maintenance, repair, and health hazards, it may actually save you money. The following are some points to consider when choosing flooring, and after you read this section, I know you will not be able to resist one of these good, better, and best choices (or at least I am hoping!).

## Marble

Marble is a gorgeous choice in flooring. There are some drawbacks, however, and I recommend that you look at your lifestyle as well as your budget before pursuing marble. Like granite, marble is a mined product. There is definitely a reason these floorings are referred to as "hard surfaces." They offer no resiliency, are cold underfoot, and are noisy in comparison to other types of floors. Did you know you can install heating under the floor to make it toasty warm? Not a cheap investment for sure, but a nice option for those whose budget will allow it. Marble is also one of the most expensive floorings. In my case, it was beyond my budget. In addition, marble can be tricky to clean and maintain. This may not be the most practical choice if you have kids running around. As a natural stone product, marble doesn't come with a warranty. When installed properly, however, it will last a lifetime.

While marble is durable and hard, granite is even more so. This characteristic must be considered in its application.

*Environmentally friendly:* Marble is all natural and does not outgas.

*Maintenance:* Marble is generally low maintenance, although some types easily stain, and these stains can be difficult to remove. For general cleaning, you must use a gentle cleaner highly diluted with water so you don't harm the marble. It is porous and easily damaged. A mild solution of borax (found in most health food stores) and warm water does the trick. You need to watch the ingredients in cleaners designed specifically for marble because many contain chemicals.

*Durability:* It is hard—it is rock and can last forever if installed properly.

*Scratch resistance:* Because of its hardness, marble cannot be scratched.

*Fire resistance:* It will not burn.

*Water resistance:* Water will not damage it.

*Installation:* Marble requires a strong subfloor.

## Ceramic Tile

Many houses built in the past decade feature ceramic tile, which is a terrific flooring choice. There is a wide range of beautiful tiles to choose from—some even mimic the look of other flooring, such as marble, granite, slate, or etched concrete. Ceramic tile flooring is one of the safest types to install. Here are its features:

*Environmentally friendly:* It is completely inert, made from natural materials, so there is no outgassing of toxic materials. Using safe grout is the main precaution required.

*Maintenance:* Sweeping and mopping with a nontoxic cleaner is all you need. No waxing, sanding, or finishing necessary. Now that is a time and cost saver!

*Durability:* It will outlast most other flooring if properly installed.

*Scratch resistance:* It will not cut or tear like other flooring.

*Fire resistance:* It will not burn.

*Water resistance:* It does not permit accumulation of water, so common spills are not a concern.

*Installation:* It is labor intensive, which means it can be expensive.

## Hardwood

Hardwood flooring is durable and safe, depending on how it is installed and maintained. I suggest buying prefinished hardwood floor tiles that have a baked-on finish. There are several types on the market. I recommend hardwood that comes in 6-inch squares held together with wire or the new self-locking floors. With these, you can avoid the glue that is commonly needed with the 12-inch squares. The following are features of hardwood flooring:

*Environmentally friendly:* It is less toxic than synthetic materials as long as toxic glues or finishes are not used.

*Maintenance:* Maintaining hardwood flooring can be more labor intensive than for ceramic tiles.

*Durability:* It is extremely long lasting. You can refinish and recoat hardwood several times without having to replace it.

*Water resistance:* Moisture can damage hardwood. Wet mopping is not recommended, and liquid spills should be cleaned up immediately.

*Installation:* Nailing, stapling, or self-locking is advised over the gluing or floating installation methods; both of the latter involve toxic glues that can outgas for long periods.

There are some "cons" that you need to take into consideration and research before purchasing wood flooring. Some new technologies have eliminated the need for waxing wood floors; however, such flooring contains chemicals that can be toxic when inhaled over the long term.

## Vinyl

Vinyl is probably the most common flooring and the one with which you are most familiar. Today, there is a wide variety of designs and colors that can really add to the look of a room. These are the features of vinyl:

*Environmentally hazardous:* A variety of chemicals are found in synthetic flooring, and the adhesives used in installation add to its toxicity.

*Maintenance:* Floor polish, which is toxic, must be applied regularly, though there are some no-wax vinyl floorings.

*Durability:* Much less durable than natural materials, vinyl will definitely not outlast ceramic tile or hardwood. Expect to replace it once or twice over the life of your house, depending on traffic and use. It is also more subject to dents, cuts, or gouges, which have to be repaired (not in sections but the entire thing!).

*Installation:* The higher quality requires professional installation. Avoid the cheap, peel-and-stick tiles, which have toxic adhesive and are less durable.

Vinyl flooring may appear to be less expensive in terms of the initial outlay of money. When you consider that it emits toxic fumes and will have to be replaced more frequently, however, it may not really save you money. What about doctor bills if it makes you or a family member sick? Investing in high-quality, durable flooring from natural materials can prevent this and adds to the resale value of your home.

## Pergo

Pergo flooring has increased in popularity and is being sold as a less expensive, scratch-resistant alternative to hardwood. It is important to remember that pergo is a synthetic material and contains the same substances as laminate countertops: paper and wood pieces bonded together with chemicals—formaldehyde and PVCs (polyvinyl chlorides, or toxic chlorinated chemicals). Pergo flooring surely outgasses these chemicals, which, as mentioned previously, are carcinogenic and mutagenic.

It is unbelievable that some environmental publications advertise Pergo. Recycling wood to conserve trees is a nice idea but not if it is making people sick. Faux wood can never be as safe or as durable as natural materials. Consumers have reported it peeling after six months. Ultimately, you get what you pay for. I will never be convinced that any synthetic can outdo Mother Nature!

## Other Flooring

Other flooring materials, such as cork and bamboo, are advertised as being more environmentally safe than vinyl. Make sure that you fully explore how the material is treated and has to be maintained before you conclude that it is actually safe. You can also obtain a sample and test it yourself to see if anyone in the house is sensitive. Bamboo appears to be a safer alternative, but it is generally treated with a polyurethane finish, which can cause health problems. Never trust that a product is safe without doing your research.

If safer alternatives are out of the question in terms of price, vinyl or laminate flooring may be tolerated better than carpeting. Vinyl is not ideal, but it may be the lesser of two evils. Wall-to-wall carpeting is always the worst choice. Some individuals with multiple chemical sensitivities have found relief of symptoms by removing the carpeting and installing vinyl with lower VOCs, safer adhesive, and a postinstallation sealant to inhibit outgassing. As one of my girlfriends said, "You won't realize how well you weren't breathing until you get rid of your carpet."

## Good, Better, Best:  Flooring

**Good:**   If you cannot replace your current floors with better flooring, clean with a nontoxic, non-corrosive agent.

**Better:**   Add better air filtration/purification to the room to help detoxify your air.

**Best:**   Replace your flooring with hardwood, ceramic tile, or other environmentally safe flooring; use only nontoxic cleaners on your new floor.

# Ventilation and Air Quality

If you do not want to invest in an individual air purifier for the living and dining rooms, it is reasonable to simply move one from another room of the house to these rooms when you are entertaining. Since these rooms usually do not have a door, the air purifier is going to be less effective, but it will still provide some benefit. You may especially want it in case someone comes over wearing some noxious perfume. If guests are going to be smoking (no longer in my house!), you may not want to run the air purifier at all, depending on the type of unit. Most filtering media will become saturated in a brief period by cigarette smoke and have to be replaced. It may be better to wait until the smokers leave and then run the unit. Air purifiers rather than air filters can be beneficial in this instance (see chapter 2).

If you have decided that these rooms can be less environmentally safe than the rest of the house because they are used less, there are simple things you can do to minimize the hazardous effects.

Close off the air circulation between this area and the rest of the house by closing the vents when it is not being used. This prevents any outgassing from moving into the rest of the house. Put a natural fabric cover over furniture that has synthetic fabrics or filling. Do not fall asleep on synthetic fabric furniture. (Gee, is your company that boring?) Avoid the use of toxic cleaners, especially oily, petroleum-based furniture polishes. For a full discussion of air quality and what to do about it, see chapter 2.

## Good, Better, Best: **Ventilation and Air Quality**

**Good:** Partially close off the vents in this room so that the outgassing from the room does not spread throughout your home.

**Better:** Don't use toxic cleaners and be sure to clean more often.

**Best:** Bring an air purifier into the room when it is in use and try to air out the room on a regular basis.

## Better Choice Mom Recommends

The following companies offer formaldehyde tests so you can check your air for outgassing:

- AllergyBuyersClub.com: www.allergybuyersclub.com; 800-789-0419

- Air Quality Sciences, Inc.: www.aqs.com; 800-789-0419

# *Furnishings*

If you shop for more environmentally safe furniture for the living/dining area, you will find that your choices are limited and that there is a lot of confusion and contradiction about what is safe and what is not. Restricting your choices to solid wood, natural fabrics, and chemically untreated material excludes most retailers. Some claim ("claim" being the key word here) to have eco-friendly furniture when in fact it is not truly chemical free.

Many companies are committed to saving the environment, so they are using recycled wood in their furniture. This is a great idea, but if the wood was previously treated with chemicals or the companies treat the wood with fungicides, petroleum-based finishes, or other toxic materials, these are not good choices for the house.

There is now furniture made from recycled plastic and other materials. What have we learned about plastics? Plastics are toxic the first time around, so it isn't a good idea (in fact, it is a terrible idea) to recycle them, add more chemicals, and then put them back in our homes a second time. (I believe in recycling and buy water in recycled bottles but would never consider buying furniture made of recycled or precycled material that outgasses chemical toxins.) Many of the additives in plastics are persistent chemicals that will not break down. The plastics are still going to outgas toxic chemicals, even if they have been used for several years and are recycled.

It can be frustrating to try to create a fashion statement when your choices are limited. You have to decide which is more important: safer indoor air and reducing your chemical exposure or appearance. For me, environmental safety is not a choice—it is a must.

The following are substances and materials to avoid in furniture:

- particleboard with urea or formaldehyde glues
- furniture made from nylon, PVC, petroleum-based products, or other chemicals
- upholstered furniture
- foam or plastic-filled furniture
- laminated finishes
- fire-proofing or fire retardants of any kind
- stain-resistant treatments

## Environmentally Safe Versus Human Safe

It can be exhausting to educate yourself about human-friendly and environmentally safe products. To add to the difficulty, there is much misinformation and confusion about what truly makes a safe product.

Unfortunately, a controversy exists over whether products that are considered safe for the environment are safe for humans too. These are not always one and the same. Many people are not informed of the harmful health effects of certain chemicals on humans, and, while they are sincere in their intent to save the environment, many of the products they use in seeming support of that goal are toxic to humans. Since your health and environment are a concern, here are a couple examples of how one may not complement the other:

- *Plastic:* You purchase water in a plastic bottle; when you are finished, rather than toss it into the garbage to go to a landfill where it will not decompose, you recycle. That recycled plastic will now be used in particleboard along with other toxic chemicals. Once it is a finished product (such as a cabinet, a dresser, or a drawer) and in your home, those toxic chemicals will outgas for the life of the product.

- *Wood:* To save the forest, you decide to purchase a synthetic wood floor. You have done your part in "saving the forest," but now you have brought a product into your home that is toxic, since "faux" wood floors consist of wood chips, straw, and chemicals made to look like wood.

For me, it does not make sense to try to save the earth at the expense of our health. There have to be solutions that do both—save the environment and protect human health. Scientists, manufacturers, and ecologists are going to have to go back to the drawing board on this one!

Another trend in recycling is poly wood, a wood substitute. Here is how poly wood is made: start with a touch of additives, add a pinch of foaming compounds, stir in an extrusion pigment system, and slowly add UV inhibitors (to prevent the product from fading after light exposure). These are all toxic chemicals. You cannot create a product that does not rot or warp and is moisture resistant without using toxic chemicals. It is a nice idea to try to reduce the contents of our landfills, but these new poly woods are processed and saturated with toxic soup. I would definitely want to see testing done before I would even consider introducing a product such as this into my home.

As mentioned throughout the book, particleboard is not advisable in the home. Whether it is made from wood chips or straw, it has to be synthetically treated to make the pieces stick together. I do not trust that the binding agents are safe since the chemicals used are not strictly regulated or tested for safety. Manufacturers are making claims without evidence to back them up. You have to read the marketing claims with a critical eye. The promotion touting that a product is "environmentally responsible" does not mean "human safe." When I started my journey of discovery, I didn't know how to ask the right questions. I believed the signs in the store that said "natural" and never thought to ask anything more. If I did ask a salesperson on the floor a question, I just accepted what he or she said rather than digging deeper. When someone tells me that a product is safe, I have learned to ask, Safe from what? Or safe for whom? Or safer compared to what?

You have to get very specific when you ask questions. Ask about the raw materials in a product. Ask about the treatments used and the steps involved in manufacturing. You also have to find the right person, the one who can truly answer your questions. The floor salesperson may not be the right one to ask since his or her goal is to make a sale, not to help you make the right choice for your home. More good questions to ask are, What materials are used in the product? and What are they treated with to make them mold resistant or flame resistant?

For a chemically sensitive person, trusting a salesperson and bringing home a product that will outgas toxic chemicals can mean a trip to the emergency room. Seeing around the hype is something I still struggle with. I would much rather believe people care about what they say and do. Since that is not necessarily the case, I have gotten quite skilled at asking the right questions—and you will too! And, oh, the power you will feel knowing that you know what the heck you are talking about!

Now that you know what can be hidden in an "environmentally safe" couch, I need to recommend again that you limit yourself to natural, solid-wood furniture that is untreated. In doing this, you still need to make sure that the product is not treated with sealants, fungicides, flame retardants, or other chemicals. Companies such as Heart of Vermont have been specializing in producing these types of products for years. Another option is to buy antique furniture. If it is old enough and of good quality, you can find hardwood that is safe since chemical treatments for wood and furniture are relatively new advances. Antiques can be expensive, but if you are patient and shop around, you can find good buys, and making a good deal is half the fun!

If you like a more modern look rather than country-style solid wood, furniture with iron or stainless steel is an option. Avoid aluminum; it has been linked to Alzheimer's disease. Several companies offer attractive, modern-style metal furniture with glass or natural materials such as canvas. There is some suggestion that metals should be avoided in beds since they can carry an electric current to which you do not want to be exposed while you are sleeping.

## Better Choice Mom Recommends

For environmentally safe furniture:

- Shaker Workshops: 415-669-7256

- SOFA U Love: 310-207-2540

- Willsboro Wood Products: 800-342-3373

- Bright Future Futon: 505-268-9738

- Heart of Vermont: 800-639-4123

## Furniture Fabrics and Cushions

If you don't want to replace your furniture, you can replace the fabric and cushions. Depending on what the frame is made of and how old it is, it may have outgassed and no longer be a significant source of chemical exposure. To be sure, you can purchase formaldehyde test kits that test the air as well as spot-test specific furniture. The spot tests are useful in determining which objects in the home may be contributing the most chemicals to the air. You simply put a drop of solution on furniture, carpeting, and mattresses. A color change shows significant levels. Testing provides a way to make more informed choices as to which items to replace.

Formaldehyde is not the only chemical that may be present in furniture cushions or fabric. As discussed in the previous chapter, Scotchgard was determined to be carcinogenic yet was still used, so more than likely your furniture may still contain it. There also may be other treatments, such as mold retardants, flame retardants, or stain-resistant chemicals. Replacing this material is important considering the fact that you may be sitting or lying on a couch for hours at a time with your skin touching this material. You can purchase organically grown cotton upholstery fabric for chairs, couches, couch cushions, curtains, or any other use.

## Better Choice Mom Recommends

For safer fabrics and cushions for furniture:

- The Cotton Place: 800-451-8866

- Janice Corp.: 800-526-4237

- Karen's Nontoxic Products: 410-378-4936

- The Living Source: 800-662-8787

## Good, Better, Best: **Furnishings**

**Good:** Find out what is in your furniture and what it was treated with so you are aware of what is and isn't toxic and you can decide what needs to stay and what can go. Choose a non-toxic cleaner. Smaller items, such as throws, rugs, and pillows, can be put out in the sun to speed the outgassing and keep those chemicals out of your indoor air.

**Better:** Re-cover furniture with a safer, nontoxic fabric and cushions.

**Best:** Replace furniture with all-natural and toxic-free furniture.

# *Decorating*

If a safe, healthy home is a priority for you, minimizing dust is another issue to consider when decorating. A minimalist approach is the way to go. The more you have on display, the more opportunity there is for dust collection and the more work it is to maintain. Many people have bottles of liquor displayed on top of a credenza or other furniture, and it takes no time for the bottles to become covered in dust. I prefer to keep other decorative items, such as pieces of crystal or figurines, in glass-enclosed types of furniture. This cuts down on dust and reduces the chance of breakage as well. Another dust collector is dried flower arrangements, some of which are also sprayed with chemicals, used as table centerpieces or displayed on shelves. A better choice is a natural beeswax candle, a piece of crystal, or an art sculpture.

Some people like to leave place mats or a tablecloth on the table. Can you imagine the dust that has gathered by the time you seat guests at this place setting! Leaving these items on your table is a no-no unless you wash linens regularly and particularly before you dine.

## Good, Better, Best:  **Decorating**

**Good:**    Keep items in glass-enclosed cases.

**Better:**  Minimize! Cut back on knickknacks altogether.

**Best:**    Decorate with natural products, such as beeswax or crystal.

# *Better Choice Mom Wisdom*

I grew up with a living room and dining room, so ridding myself of those rooms and using the space for a game room and an office instead is a 180-degree change from where I started. If you would have told me 10 years ago that I would no longer have my pig collection or a formal living room, I would have thought, "That's impossible!" Today, as I look at how easily life flows and how great we feel, I cannot imagine it any other way. My son may never know what a Magnavox hi-fi is, but he will know the joys of playing with his friends in the game room and knowing that mom is near. I hope that the clear, uncluttered environment that I have created will help him avoid some of the distractions that I had.

Though replacing carpeting, furniture, upholstery, and decorations with more natural products is expensive, it may prevent future health problems and such items usually last longer. Each piece of furniture that is emitting chemicals contributes to the total load of stress on your body. This strains the body's ability to detoxify and deal with everyday chemicals. Every change that you can make in the home to reduce your chemical exposure makes a difference in how you think and feel. And I am here to tell you that you can create a beautiful atmosphere without adding toxic chemicals. By implementing some of the good choices and then letting some time pass, you will become more comfortable with some better choices and then move on to the best choices. Things that are worth it and the most rewarding take time. Give yourself that time. Remember, the world was not created in a day!

# CHAPTER 8

# The Bedroom

## Don't Let the Bedbugs Bite

Only I can change my life. No one can do it for me.
—Carol Burnett

IT'S AMAZING HOW THE EVERYDAY STRESSES, fears, and anxieties of life that can leave you emotionally depleted and physically ill can quickly overtake your life to the point of invading your most private sanctuary and protective environment: the bedroom. I was stressed, depressed, and ill after I realized that my poor choices were the link to David's asthma, skin rashes, and multiple chemical sensitivities. Those feelings hung over me like a dark cloud wherever I went, and I could not shake them even when I knew I needed to give myself permission for a "time-out." I vividly recall how violated I felt by the myths and lies that bombarded me through television and magazines advertisements with regard to the products I brought into my home. Without being aware of it, I began to retreat into my bedroom, hoping that it would all "go away" yet knowing that it was up to me to deal with it and take charge if David was ever going to be well.

Fear took over my subconscious, and without my realizing it, hours spent in the bedroom became days. As I tore up my kitchen and bathrooms, my bedroom was my safe harbor, or so I thought. As I pushed my body and mind to learn what had brought about the collapse of my world, I would fall asleep most nights with book and highlighter in hand, only to wake a few hours later and go back to my research.

I was obsessed with reading about the chemicals and toxins that invaded my home. Medical reference material, magazines, old newspaper articles, and correspondence from the people whom I was reaching out to for answers had gone from cluttering my kitchen counter, dining room table, and family room floor to being stacked in piles on my dresser. Boxes of literature lined the walls of my bedroom. Papers were piled high on the bed where there had once been decorative pillows. Books lying all over the floor were tagged, highlighted, and sticky-noted in the hope that they would help me understand what was happening to what I thought was my safe, impenetrable world at home. Since I thought I was a "bad sleeper," I just accepted the miserable way I felt in the morning and how sluggish I felt by 3:00 P.M. All the signs of depression were present, but with David's illness and all the changes I was making, I brushed them aside. I stopped eating in the kitchen because it was easier to eat a sandwich or a bowl of cereal while I sat on my bed reading.

David lay next to me at night because it was easier that way to tend to him during the night rather than to keep running down the hall to comfort him. Plus, with my new understanding of all the chemicals that surrounded us, I began to feel paranoid that something awful would happen during the night, so the sound of him still breathing gave me comfort. I look back on these memories and am struck by the way I was living and how I was really losing my grip. I was sinking without even knowing I was drowning. I think this happens to us more often than we think. We tread water, just going through the motions of living, and then wake up one day to find ourselves so disconnected from other people and the "real" world that oftentimes we cannot find our way back.

One night, I was awakened by David's whimpers of pain, caused by his red, blotchy, swollen skin. In absolute exhaustion, I looked around my bedroom and was shocked at what I saw. It was as if I saw it for the first time, and I was stunned. How did this happen? I had been so "sucked down" into a black hole that I didn't have the power to dig myself out of it. How could I ever get through this and fight this? There were books, boxes, papers, blankets, pillows, dirty glasses and plates, fast-food wrappers, and clothes scattered all over this small room, with David and I parked in the middle. I said to myself, "What am I doing? I've spent hours organizing and detoxing my house, only to retreat to the one room I haven't; and even worse, I brought all those nasty things into the room, exposing David to just what I thought I had taken out of my home." It was no wonder he did not have a good night's sleep. The junk food wrappers (let alone the food!), the chemically laden newspapers, and the pillows were all toxic! I had gotten so bogged down by frustrations and fear that my vision was no longer clear.

I found David's wagon and began to load up the books and papers and unbury myself physically, mentally, and emotionally. I stripped the bed, threw the sheets in the wash, and opened the windows. David and I lay on the stripped bed, no longer surrounded by my books and work. As the cool air blew in, I was taken away into a deep sleep. They say everything looks brighter in the morning, and I can say that I woke with a new sense of strength, a clearer head, and a huge question (that still weighs on my mind on bad days): What would David and I be like today if I had made different choices before he was born and he had never gotten sick?

From this story you can see that the bedroom is probably one of the most important rooms in the house for me. It was my place for safe rejuvenation. When I saw what I had done to my sanctuary in pursuit of protecting David and me, I went at my makeover with a newfound vigor. My bedroom is the room in my house that has undergone the most visible change over the past few years.

Before David was born, my bedroom used to be a place where I would go to relax and wind down from the day. After David arrived, because of his illness, my room became a place of pent-up stress, anxiety, and anguish (which, I learned, I was passing on to him). I didn't realize that this was part of the reason why sleep was something I could not manage. Today, getting a good night's sleep is not a problem, though it has taken me quite a few years to provide my body with and allow my mind a sleep zone. Because of my own battle with this, I have taught my son to be a great sleeper. I am still making changes today to continue my efforts to provide my body and mind with what they need.

The first thing I began to see in my bedroom journal was all the things that I did in my bedroom, with sleep being way down on the list of priorities. Odd, since aren't the bed, pillows, and pajamas for sleeping? What was staring me in the face were all the activities that went on there: running on my treadmill, watching television, reading a book, finishing paperwork, folding laundry, eating, and writing my "to do" list for the next morning. So many things happened in my bedroom that my brain never switched off; it was always in an activity mode.

Today when I enter my bedroom, I automatically relax. My room today is set up for unwinding and beginning the process of sleep. I find that I require less sleep because I get to sleep faster and sleep more soundly than I did before. I feel good in the morning and want to get out of bed to start my day.

The bedroom should serve the function it was designed for, and that is a safe haven and a place to become reenergized (no, not like the Energizer bunny, who keeps on going). Sleep is an important time for the body to rest and heal itself. It is a good idea to make this your safest room in the house. During sleep, if your stomach is empty, your liver has a chance to detoxify chemicals to which you have been exposed during the day. If your bedroom has a lot of chemicals, then your body has to work overtime. Why not give it a break and make your bedroom human and earth friendly?

If you consider that all day long we are exposed to chemicals outside the home that we cannot control, you need to have a room that is your "safety net," where your body is not being challenged. How can that happen if there are chemicals outgassing in your bedroom and the place is a gym, an office, and a utility room? It is worth the effort to discover what health hazards may be in the bedroom and to create the best environment (defining space again) for your body to rest in.

## The Bedroom Journal

Is your bedroom a place where you can relax? If restful sleep is your priority, ideally there should be very little in your bedroom except a bed and maybe a night table with a lamp. That is it! People who have difficulty falling or staying asleep may not realize that having too many activities in this room can contribute to poor sleep. It sends a message to your subconscious that the bed is also for other activities. Think about it: If your bills, paperwork, homework, or other clutter is on or around your bed, it is like background noise that can prevent you from relaxing. The more stuff and clutter you have in your bedroom, the more it distracts you from the real purpose of the room—sleep.

There are some people who like doing household activities in the bedroom. If that is the way you want to define your bedroom, that is fine, but then you need to ask whether the room is designed for that. If it is, there are still things you can do to make it more aesthetic, more functional, and less distracting to sleep. Since I have a tendency to overwork my brain, I have what I call "God's Book." Before I go to sleep, I write down all the stresses and anxieties that are on my mind and as a result have little trouble sleeping through the night, knowing that my problems are in good hands.

My bedroom is the only place in my house where I can use my treadmill without disturbing others, so I needed a way to show myself the difference between exercising and sleeping. I moved my treadmill to one side of the room and put a beautiful room divider in front of it. This way, when I walk into the room, I do not see a huge eyesore and my brain does not think exercise, so the treadmill's presence does not interfere with my sleep mode. When I walk around the divider, the treadmill is facing the window so I can see outdoors while running. I have no distractions and I do not see my bed, which perhaps on some days is beckoning me to return. Also, isolating the treadmill allows others to respect its purpose. David is wonderful about not coming in and interrupting when I am running because I have created boundaries for both of us.

So now it is time to take an inventory of all the activities that go on in the bedrooms in your house and what exactly is in those rooms. Assessing and reflecting on all the objects and activities in the bedroom allows you to evaluate and consider making changes to improve the bedroom environment. Answer the journal questions for each bedroom in your house.

# Journal Questions: Bedroom

### Questions to help locate toxins

1. How health friendly is my bedroom?

2. How often do I clean my bedroom?

3. What kind of cleaners do I use?

4. How often do I wash and change the sheets?

5. Do I have trouble sleeping?

6. Do I never want to get up in the morning?

7. Do I keep dirty laundry in the bedroom?

8. How many electronic items are in my bedroom?

9. Do I sleep with an electric blanket?

10. Is there any leakage at the windows or a sliding glass door?

### Questions to help organize

1. What activities take place in the bedroom? List all of them and take an inventory of the items in the room that go with each activity. For example, with "office work," you might list desk, computer, and laptop; with "watch television," you might list television, VCR, stand, and videos.

2. Whom do I share the room with (spouse, pets, kids)?

3. What physical limitations are there in my bedroom (walk-in and other closets, overhead lighting)?

4. Does my room give me mixed messages about its purpose?

5. Do others use the room? If so, are they supposed to?

■ ■ ■

I used to have a tough time getting up in the morning, but I didn't think anything was wrong. I blamed it on age, having David and dealing with his challenges, and having more people asking things from me all day long, so the fact that I was always tired was acceptable to me. For a long time I believed that feeling tired when I first woke up was normal, or I thought maybe I was depressed. Well, if you also feel this way, maybe you are not tired or depressed; maybe there is just something in the bedroom that is toxic and is causing you not to get the REM sleep you need or affecting your body in some way.

I noticed a big change in David and me just by changing to health-friendly bed and bedding. I encased the beds with mattress covers, put on all-cotton sheets, and removed the foam pillows from my bed. Within that same week, I was sleeping better and had an easier time getting up in the morning. I stopped getting up in the middle of the night, and when I woke and it was morning, I wondered where the time had gone. I now feel better rested, and putting my feet to the floor has never been easier.

Unfortunately, the bedroom is also the first area where I slip into old habits when my body is fighting off a cold or I've put in too many hours on the road. Before I know it, I'm back on the bed doing paperwork, making my "to do" list, and even making phone calls. I forget that I am doing nothing about the cold or the overwork because I am not resting or rejuvenating my body. I am just doing work lying down! Once again, I am giving my body mixed messages. To avoid this, the following are areas to address in the bedroom:

- organization
- carpeting
- beds and bedding
- window coverings
- controlling dust
- electromagnetic radiation
- closets
- special concerns for the nursery

## Organization

Get rid of clutter, especially if you cannot sleep! Remember, less is best. The less you have in the bedroom, the less chance there is for chemical outgassing, dust, and mold as well as mental/psychological stress. If space is limited in your house and you have nowhere else to put things, such as a desk, then do what I did to hide my treadmill—get a room divider. They come in different styles and actually can be decorative. Also, chests or furniture with doors on it can enhance your space visually so that you are not looking at clutter.

Do you have too many knickknacks and decorative stuff in your bedroom? For allergic individuals, dust can be a real problem. The more you have in your bedroom, the more opportunities to collect dust. This is especially true of stuffed animals. Limiting the number to 1 or 2 instead of 50 can cut down on dust. What your mind sees or smells is what it thinks about.

## Television Versus No Television

Nearly one-third of children 2 to 7 years old and nearly two-thirds of those 8 to18 years old have a television set in their bedrooms. The American Academy of Pediatrics warns that television can promote dangerous behavior in youngsters. Think of all the violence on television. A study by researchers at The Johns Hopkins University School of Medicine, along with experts from the Centers for Disease Control and the National Institutes of Health, concludes that a child's weight increases with the number of hours he or she spends watching television each day. (Don't harp about weight; just cut back television for an hour, and you might see great results.) The average child watches three hours of television a day. You have to decide if this is a healthy choice for your children, especially if you have cable and they are able to watch whatever they want with no supervision.

Another thing to remember and take into consideration for adults and children is electromagnetic radiation. You want to make sure the television is not too close to the bed, particularly if you fall asleep with the television on. Another enhancement is to place a covering over the set. Some people use a cloth similar to a table runner with a nice design that matches the room or purchase a stand that has doors that close. It hides the television and takes the focus off it so you do not have to look at a less-than-attractive blank screen.

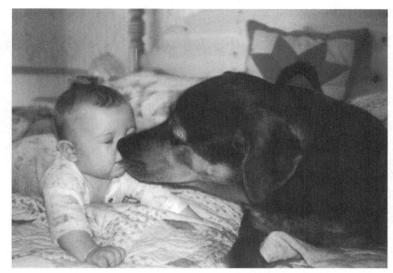

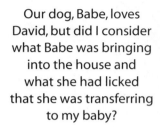

Our dog, Babe, loves David, but did I consider what Babe was bringing into the house and what she had licked that she was transferring to my baby?

## Pets Versus No Pets

If you are allergic to animal fur or dander or what pets might track in on their paws (pesticides, fertilizer), then there should be absolutely no pets in the bedroom. Believe it or not, there are people who are allergic to their animals but still insist on keeping them in the bedroom. If you just cannot bear to shut them out, then at least vacuum and change the bedding more often. Give them their own bed; place it beside yours so they are near you, and teach them to use it. Keeping your pet clean is also a must. You can wash animals with a solution from the pet store that denatures the dander and makes it less allergenic. Another thing to consider is the parasites that your pet may be carrying. Humans and animals can share their bugs back and forth, so you want to be aware. My dog is my second child, so I have two beds for him. One bed is off the kitchen so that he can be with us while David and I prepare meals, and the other is at the foot of my bed. There is no reason to replace bed linens and coverings with nontoxic products and then let a dog sleep on the bed!

## Good, Better, Best: **Organization**

**Good:** Commit to moving one thing out of the bedroom that you don't use.

**Better:** Choose only two things that you want to do in the bedroom, such as sleeping and writing letters.

**Best:** Restrict furnishings to a bed, a light, and a dresser. Take further steps by utilizing natural enhancers, such as beeswax candles, soft music, or a chaise lounge for reading.

# Carpeting

Many environmentally sensitive individuals have found relief of symptoms just by replacing carpet with natural flooring in the bedroom. As we discussed in chapter 2, carpet can outgas chemicals for years as well as collect bacteria, dust, and mold. You might experience relief of symptoms such as nasal congestion, wheezing, and restless sleep by making this change. If you are not able to replace carpeting throughout the whole house, just doing the bedroom can have a big impact. It is worth the investment.

I know getting up and stepping onto a cold floor can really be a harsh awakening, but so can a nagging headache. As I mentioned before, I am the queen of slippers! Place them beside your bed so you can jump right into them in the morning. You might also try a small decorative rug (all natural without rubber backing, please), which is also warm to the toesies!

# Beds and Bedding

The next biggest hazard in the bedroom is the bed itself. Today's mattresses are constructed with a wide variety of petrochemicals, some of the worst being vinyl and polyurethane foam. Studies with mice have shown that when you blow air over bedding or carpet and then expose mice to this air, they experience respiratory irritation and neurotoxic effects such as seizures and even death. My first step toward getting rid of the toxins was to purchase organic, 100 percent cotton encasements called barrier cloths (see appendix for where to purchase) for David's and my pillows and mattresses since I could not afford to buy new beds. I then sealed the wooden beds.

Environmental medical specialists are now theorizing that many health problems in children can be caused by or made worse from toxic chemicals in bedding. More studies will have to be done to prove this, but why not be proactive and use the safest bedding possible? Unless you have specifically sought out safe bedding, you can be sure your bed is treated with a multitude of chemicals. Do not forget about the bed frame, which can be particleboard or wood treated with pesticides. An air purifier for the room helps, as does opening the windows and even placing the bed out in the sun for a period of time to release the chemicals.

In addition to petrochemicals, flame retardants are an issue. One of the most toxic flame retardants is penta-bromo-dephenyl ether. Some scientists and environmentalists are calling for a ban on this chemical. It has been found in fish, wildlife, and humans around the globe. It is showing up in breast milk in high concentrations. My question is, What usually kills or injures people in a fire? Smoke! Do flame retardants really save lives? Is it justifiable to poison ourselves daily for something that may never happen? This is a very personal choice, but now you have the knowledge to make a more informed decision.

The fact that this chemical is showing up in breast milk is disturbing enough, but another sad issue is that this chemical is persistent, meaning it does not break down quickly, remains in the environment, and is stored in our body fat. Even if it is banned, millions of pounds of persistent chemicals will remain in our soil, water, and air for generations to come.

Most department stores simply do not carry organic bedding, so it is necessary to purchase it through reputable mail order houses (do your research here, too). Most of the sheets and bedding in stores are treated with chemicals such as pesticides, mold retardants, flame retardants, and more. Fabrics are sprayed to prevent mold during shipping. Polyester and synthetics are chemically treated. Wrinkle-resistant fabrics are also very toxic. Again, how many parties have you had where people want to come see your sheets? And I was wondering why I could not sleep? It is amazing that anybody wakes up rested! Do not panic, though; there are companies that make all-organic and 100 percent cotton bedding and clothes (see appendix for sources). Believe it or not, you have to get a doctor's prescription in order to buy mattresses with no flame retardant. If your doctor will not write a prescription for you, there are physicians who specialize in environmental medicine who will help you. You can obtain a list of physicians through the American Academy of Environmental Medicine (see appendix).

A word on water beds: Get rid of them. There is no way around it—they are bad news. The vinyl is loaded with chemicals, and they may outgas for years.

## Good, Better, Best: **Beds and Bedding**

**Good:** Air the mattress out in the sun for a day and vacuum the mattress front and back. Commit to using new chemical-free linens. If you cannot change the bed or bedding, ozonate the bed and bedding and get an air purifier to handle chemical outgassing.

**Better:** Encase the mattress and pillows. Buy a new organic pillow. Seal the wood (see chapters 2 and 3 on sealing cabinets).

**Best:** Get all-organic, untreated mattresses, furniture, and bedding.

## Window Coverings

Other sources of toxins to consider are miniblinds or other window coverings. Many are made from vinyl and other synthetic material treated with chemicals.

Dusting blinds helps cut down on dust. Lightweight curtains from natural fabrics that can be washed are an option as well. Depending on the view from your window (or the potential view in!), no covering is also something to consider. Simplicity can be attractive, so consider something like a silk valance to frame the window.

## Controlling Dust

The first thing to consider in controlling dust is, the less stuff you have in the room, the better. Get rid of carpeting and clutter. The next issue is, clean often! Again, the less you have, the less you have to clean. Dust mites live off human dead skin and can collect in the pillows and mattress. People with allergies are often told to get dust covers to help with this problem, but what they often end up getting are toxic, plastic-type covering. Bad choice! Again, barrier cloths are great for controlling dust as they are easy to put on and take off and can be washed as needed. Headboards with shelving units at the head of the bed are just opportunities for dust and clutter to collect—another definite no-no. A room air purifier can also help control dust.

How often you clean has an impact on the air quality of the room. You have to determine how much cleaning is best for you. For instance, I have to clean David's room more often than I do mine. He and I read together in his bedroom at night, and Babe, our dog, joins us. David also has sleep-overs, and, as you know, boys seem to be little dirt magnets. My bedroom, on the other hand, stays relatively clean. I no longer clean on a specific day but instead do it when and where it is needed.

---

## Good, Better, Best:  **Dust Control**

**Good:**　The less clutter, the better. If you cannot wash your bedding (duvet, comforter, or bedspread), fluff it in the dryer. If you must have curtains and they are not 100 percent cotton, go for a light fabric that can be washed.

**Better:**　Clean as often as the room needs it, particularly if you have a pet or the bedroom is also used for a playroom for your child and his or her friends.

**Best:**　No knickknacks, no shelved headboards, no storage under the bed. Be sure to dust under and behind the bed.

---

## Better Choice Mom Recommends

The ideal "safe" bedroom looks like this:

- hardwood floor (not treated with chemicals)
- all-natural furniture
- organic mattress, pillow, and bedding with no flame retardants
- air purifier
- minimal doodads!

# *Electromagnetic Radiation*

As mentioned in the discussion about television, it is important to pay attention to electromagnetic fields (EMFs) in the bedroom. If you sleep with a clock, radio, television, computer, or other appliance plugged in right behind or under your bed, the current may be too close to your body. The EMF could be affecting you negatively. You can get devices to measure the amount of radiation, but prevention is prudent. It is best to plug in appliances farther away from the bed. Just this simple adjustment can have a dramatic effect on your sleep.

An alarm clock that plugs into the wall emits an EMF of 5 to 10 milligauss up to two feet away. This means if it is within arm's reach, you are being exposed to its radiation. Battery-operated clocks are much safer; their electromagnetic field is negligible. If the power goes out, you also have the benefit of the clock being unaffected so you will wake up on time. Once again, less is better. Anything electric that is unnecessary in the bedroom should be removed. By now you have likely guessed that an electric blanket is an absolute no-no, particularly if you are pregnant. (Studies have shown that EMFs from blankets can cause over 80 percent of problem pregnancies.) If you insist on having an electric blanket or are caring for someone who is elderly, turn the electric blanket on until it reaches the desired temperature. Then turn it off and unplug it from the wall.

## Good, Better, Best: **EMFs**

**Good:** All electrical items should be four to six feet away from your head.

**Better:** Unplug any electrical items not in use and use them with batteries if you can.

**Best:** Limit the number of electrical items to "necessary only" and keep them a safe distance from the bed. Get rid of the electric blanket. Turn off the electric current from outlets behind your bed with a kill switch at the wall.

# Closets

Are your closets a disorganized nightmare? Many people have no real idea how to organize clothes. Everything is all mixed up. Have you ever looked in your closet (where you have tons of clothes) and complained, "I have nothing to wear?" It is probably because you simply cannot find what you want, or it is too crowded to see. Sorting through what you really wear and getting rid of what you do not is very liberating. You may need to invite a friend to help you since many times we hang on to things for emotional reasons. A good rule is, If I have not worn it in the past six months or longer, out it goes. You know the saying: Get rid of the old to make room for the new.

Though you may think this is an aesthetic issue, the closet can be another source of chemical outgassing in your home. Most clothes and shoes are made from synthetic materials, which are treated with chemicals. Some sensitive individuals would benefit from removing clothing and shoes and placing them in a different closet in the house if space permits. You can also treat clothes and shoes with ozone by opening the closet door and letting an ozone generator run for a few hours. Then keep the closet door closed while you are sleeping.

Dust also builds up in closets. People get lazy when they vacuum and never do the closet. Again, no carpet is best, but if you do have carpet, you should vacuum in the closet every time you do the room. It is best not to store things on the floor of the closet so you can clean it more easily.

Do not put dirty laundry in your closet. The clothes you wear absorb pollution, chemicals, odors, your sweat, and who knows what else. You do not need your dirty clothes incubating stink in the closet right next to your clean clothes. It just does not make any sense. Laundry chutes that go directly to the laundry room are great if you have a two-story house.

Train family members to take their clothes immediately to the laundry room after they take them off. It may sound like "just another thing to do" and even a bit odd, but after you develop the habit, you find it is very easy and much nicer than having to go around and collect dirty clothes from all over the house. If that does not work for you, at least have a clothes hamper somewhere besides in the bedroom. Some people use the bathroom, though I personally do not want the stinky stuff in that room, either, since it is where I go to get clean. You need to figure out what works for you and your family. The obvious place for the clothes hamper is the laundry room. That is what the room is designed for.

## Closet Air Fresheners

Some people like to use potpourri or stick-on air fresheners in their closets. If you consider how these work and what they are doing, that does not make good sense either. My first question is, Why should the closet need it in the first place? If the closet does need an air freshener, what is causing the odor in the closet? When you find the source of the odor, get rid of it! If you keep the dirty laundry elsewhere and dust or clean regularly, you should not need an air freshener. Get rid of the source of the problem; do not just try to cover it up.

Air fresheners do not "freshen" the air. They use synthetic chemicals to mask an offensive odor and interfere with our ability to smell. These chemicals coat the nasal passages with an undetectable oil film or deaden our nerves to the smell. You may like the immediate result of the supposedly fresh smell, but have you considered the damage it may be causing your body?

If you insist on adding pleasant smells, use essential oils or herbal sachets that are not treated with chemicals, as are most potpourri. You can use old socks and nylons filled with dried flowers and oils and hang them in the closet or put them in the dresser drawer. You can use dried lavender in small muslin bags, which is a simple, inexpensive, and all-natural solution. Once you experience natural products such as high-quality essential oils versus synthetic chemicals, your tastes and preferences will change dramatically. You will find that air fresheners and synthetic fragrance you once liked are now offensive.

## Mothballs

While most people use mothballs only in basements, attics, and storage containers, it is important to say right here that mothballs are an absolute no in bedroom closets. Two different chemicals that can be in mothballs make them harmful: naphthalene and paradichlorobenzene. There are a number of reasons why you do not want these chemicals anywhere in your house, much less in your bedroom.

Exposure to naphthalene can cause systemic reactions, including nausea, headache, profuse sweating, hematuria (blood in the urine), fever, anemia, liver damage, vomiting, convulsions, and coma. It can also cause eye irritation, confusion, excitement, malaise, abdominal pain, irritation to the bladder, jaundice, renal shutdown, and dermatitis. Poisoning can result from ingestion of large doses, skin and/or eye contact, inhalation, or skin absorption.

Paradichlorobenzene is a white solid crystal with a wet oily surface. It is extremely volatile, giving off a strong penetrating odor. Paradichlorobenzene is commonly found in mothballs, moth crystals, and diaper, toilet, and room deodorizers. Inhalation can result in headache, swollen eyes, stuffy head, loss of appetite, nausea, vomiting, and throat and eye irritation. Allergies and skin irritation have been reported with prolonged skin contact. Symptoms from ingestion include nausea, vomiting, diarrhea, liver and kidney damage, and methemoglobianemia (which interferes with the uptake of oxygen). Good grief!

Do you want to poison yourself and the environment just to protect your clothes? Do you want to take a small potential problem and create a larger, more dangerous one? Do you have small children who could be poisoned if they got hold of mothballs, thinking that they were candy? A bigger question for those clotheshorses: Are you holding on to clothes that should be "out of here" anyway? Worse yet, do you really want to walk around reeking of "eau de mothballs"? Herbs such as lavender, wormwood, and rosemary are natural moth repellents, and they smell absolutely wonderful (see appendix for recipe).

## Good, Better, Best: **Closets**

**Good:** Don't overstock your closet. Many clothes and shoes are synthetic and thus are continually outgassing. Keep your closet doors closed.

**Better:** Don't use any spray air fresheners, mothballs, or synthetic chemical fragrances.

**Best:** Vacuum the closet regularly. Do not keep dirty clothes in the closet. Use naturally scented sachets and moth repellants. Keep toxic clothes, such as new or dry-cleaned clothing, out of the bedroom until washed or aired out.

# *Special Concerns for the Nursery*

Children's needs in the bedroom are different from those of parents, and infants' bedrooms require even more attention. Whereas you might have priorities such as romance for adults (I bet you were wondering if I would ever mention that!) and play areas for toddlers, the most important issue in the nursery is safety and promoting good health.

You want your baby to sleep in an environment that is as chemical free as possible. The crib is probably the most important purchase you will make, with the mattress and bedding a very close second. Cribs should be all-natural wood that is untreated, and the mattress and bedding need to be 100 percent all-organic cotton material with no flame retardant. This applies to sheets, blankets, and mattress as well as pajamas and stuffed animals.

Children's bodies and their immune systems do not have as many detoxifying enzymes as adults' do. This means that chemical outgassing has a much more dramatic impact on them. Infants' organs and systems, especially the brain and nervous system, are still developing after birth. The brain can be permanently damaged by pesticides and other neurotoxins. That is why it is dangerous not to know what is in the products you are using. You do not want to find out the hazards after the fact. You want to take the stance that everything is suspect or guilty until proven otherwise. You may not be able to change everything in the house right away, but I suggest a zero tolerance for chemicals in the nursery. Do not make what should be a time of growth, nurturing, and development a battle to fight off toxic chemicals and a struggle simply to breathe.

It is estimated that once we decorate and add furnishings to a room, we triple our exposure to chemical outgassing. I have mentioned these issues in other rooms, but to review and take notes for your journal or list priorities for nursery safety, consider the following:

- crib
- bedding
- carpet
- wallpaper
- paint
- air fresheners
- plastic toys
- synthetic stuffed animals
- baby wipes
- petroleum jelly

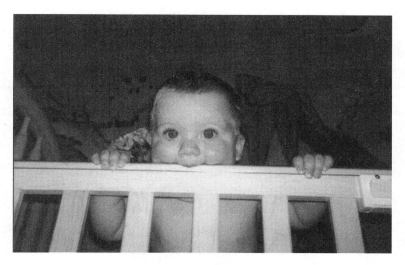

Like every baby, David chewed and sucked on everything. Now, knowing what I know about plastics and what I was cleaning his crib with … big mistake!

- baby powder with talc
- changing tables with synthetic coverings
- disposable diapers
- waterproof padding

It is hard to believe that most of the wonderful presents you receive that were purchased at department stores are toxic time bombs that can wreak havoc in the nursery. Plastic toys and teething products are the worst because children will put them in their mouth and directly absorb the chemicals. As mentioned in chapter 3, plastics are treated with a variety of chemicals, including polyvinyl chloride and other plasticizers. All plastics are a problem. That means pacifiers too. An all-natural washcloth washed in nontoxic soap and frozen is great for teething babies! It may be difficult to tell friends and family not to buy certain gifts, but if you register with companies that make safer products, it can be an opportunity to educate other parents to make better choices for their families. Cuts down on all the returns too!

## Crib Safety

Chemicals in babies' mattresses, bumpers, sheets, pajamas, and bedding have been implicated in SIDS (sudden infant death syndrome). Other causes of death in children are strangulation and suffocation from becoming wrapped up and tangled in these items. To avoid this, you need to make sure there is nothing in the crib that can hurt your baby. There should be nothing in the crib except the baby, lying on an all-natural sheet and, if you insist, covered with a light all-natural-fiber blanket, both of which have been washed in nontoxic laundry soap—no toys, no pillows, no stuffed animals, no exceptions! Remember that babies' temperatures will naturally run warmer than those of adults, so they are not as cold as we think they are. You can see how warm a baby really is by holding his or her foot.

### Better Choice Mom Recommends

For information on SIDS, see www.mercola.com/2001/jan/14/crib_death.htm.

For a product that keeps crib sheets held down tightly so infants cannot get tangled in them, see Baby Sleep Safe at www.babysleepsafe.com.

## The Importance of 100 Percent Organic Cotton

Some companies offer two choices: conventional cotton or 100 percent organic cotton. In order to be an educated consumer, you have to understand what is involved in growing and processing cotton and why you should pay more for organic. If we knew all the steps involved in producing our clothing and bedding, we would probably never buy anything but 100 percent organic. Conventional cotton crops are heavily sprayed with pesticides. In one season they can be sprayed 30 to 40 times. To put this in context, cotton represents only 3 percent of farmland yet consumes 25 percent of the pesticides. Insects are now becoming resistant to pesticides, so crops require more and more heavy spraying.

Once the cotton is made into material, processing of the fabric includes bleaching, dyeing, and multiple chemical treatments for making the fabric moth repellant, wrinkle resistant, mold resistant, flame resistant, and who knows what else we are not told. Each process adds more and more chemicals, some of which are carcinogenic. Untreated or unbleached cotton may not have had some of the chemical finishes, but it was still sprayed with pesticides.

Cotton, whether organic or not, is still better than synthetics such as polyester, which is made from petrochemicals and is non-biodegradable. So what you are buying to cover your own and your baby's precious body is saturated with cancer-causing chemicals. Now that is the truth, and I hope it scares you into action!

## Good, Better, Best:  **Cotton**

**Good:**    Use conventional cotton instead of synthetics such as polyester.

**Better:**    Use unbleached, untreated cotton (still has pesticides) and wash in nontoxic soap.

**Best:**    Use 100 percent organic, untreated cotton with no flame retardants.

## Baby Products

Get rid of petroleum jelly, baby powder, and toxic baby wipes—these "nice smelling" baby products are toxic. Once you do so, you will really see how nice your baby does smell! I remember applying petroleum jelly on David's red bottom and swollen genitals not knowing that I wasn't healing anything at all. I wasn't sure if it was better to let David stay in a wet diaper or watch him suffer through the pain of wiping, patting, rubbing, and rediapering.

Petroleum products, such as petroleum jelly, are toxic to our bodies. We have been taught to believe that petroleum jelly is safe. *Wrong.* It "seals" the skin, clogs pores, attracts dirt, and pulls essential trace minerals from the skin. Our skin does need moisture, so purchase nonpetroleum jellies and water-soluble products that are safer, more natural moisturizers (see appendix).

Baby powder contains talc, which also clogs pores and has been linked to cancer. Several companies make baby powders with more natural ingredients such as tapioca starch, which absorbs oil and moisture.

Baby wipes contain alcohol (which is drying and irritating to skin) and other synthetic chemicals and fragrances. Though there are some nonalcohol wipes, most have a fragrance, and guess what? It is synthetic! (Soapworks has recently introduced safe wipes.)

The truth is that no governmental organization is truly protecting our children. Parents need to take individual responsibility for educating themselves. Organizations that may have set out to protect the public have been affected by budget cuts, politics, pressure from industry, and, unfortunately, public apathy.

The Consumer Product Safety Commission (CPSC) was formed with the mission to protect the public against the unreasonable risk of injury and death associated with consumer products. It is surprising to learn that testing is not required before infant products are sold. The CPSC recalls products only after there have been reports of injury and death. It can take months, if not years, for a product to be recalled. Meanwhile, other injuries and deaths can occur and continue to occur. It's best to treat every product as suspect until proven safe. This means that you have to investigate and ask questions about everything.

## Better Choice Mom Wisdom

If you are like I was at this point, downright frustrated, please know that I sympathize. I just wanted to blink my eyes and have all the changes I needed to make in my home just happen. As I've said throughout this book, things of value take time. As with the other rooms in the house, make a list to decide what needs to be done first in the bedrooms and what can be done over time.

I love my bedroom, but it took me a long time to get it just so. My list of the things I wanted was a long one and included a new mattress, comforter, pillows, and encasements. I was able to get things sooner than I would have on my own by making my "wish list" known to family and friends. They pitched in to purchase a comforter for me for my birthday. My son and his father bought me my pillows. Slowly, over time, my bedroom became my safe harbor.

Little things, such as moving your alarm clock so it is away from your head and eliminating the television, can be done immediately and without any cost. Remember, as you take each step, you are making a commitment to yourself. I had to learn how to love myself and not look at my old self as a bad self. By slowly beginning to make good, better, and best choices for your family, you are saying you are worth taking care of. This will have a ripple effect—a good one—on all those around you.

---

# CHAPTER 9

# The Laundry Room
## The Never-Ending Search for the Other Sock

Better keep yourself clean and bright; you are the window through which you must see the world.
> —George Bernard Shaw

**B**EFORE WE BEGIN, one thing I would love to know is where do the socks go? This one, ladies, I am confused about and wonder if any of us will ever find the answer.

An answer I *can* help you with is how to streamline the drudgery and eliminate the toxicity of doing the laundry. We'll look at our strange need to have our cloths smell like country forests, fresh rain, and lemons. We'll discuss how white is white. And most important, we'll learn how poor choices can cause unhealthy side effects. I learned the hard way how toxic laundry products can be when I wrapped David in a freshly laundered towel or put him to bed on what I thought were the perfectly clean, unwrinkled sheets. The effect on him was almost immediate, and it wasn't nice!

Looking back on how I once used my laundry room and how I use it today, I'm struck by the many differences. The design, if you even want to call it a design, of my old laundry room was working against me. My first mistake was that I had so many products in the cabinet that I really had no idea what was even in there. I constantly complained that I didn't have enough room. Most of the products were half used since they didn't live up to their claims of brightening or removing the most stubborn of stains. With my clean freak mentality, I would even mix products in the hope that, combined, they would work! Now that I understand how combining chemicals can be so dangerous, I consider myself very lucky to be breathing.

I also bought into the great marketing ploy that clothes are not clean unless they smell like lemons or ocean breezes. Yeah, I admit it—that was me. I believed that in order for David to smell like a baby, he had to smell like fabric softener. When I was doing the wash, my whole house smelled lemon fresh, but there was nothing natural about those lemons. It was nothing but synthetic scent streaming its way through my house, and it stayed in the clothes long after I put them away, bringing that wonderful toxic scent into the bedrooms and linen closets and into our night sleep. David's reaction to his clothes came quickly after I did the laundry and was easy to spot, although in the beginning it never even dawned on me that his skin irritation could be coming from his extra-washed, softened, and fluffed cloths. David's skin was irritated most the time in his early days, and the skin problems eventually settled in behind his knees and on his stomach, arms, and cheeks. I continued to add to the poor child's misery by doubling my efforts when he stained something. I used even more chemicals to get stains out of his shirts, bibs, and diapers. My goodness, the thought of the toxins I was adding to David's and my life without realizing it makes me shiver. Cleaning faster and more furiously as David got sicker, I didn't realize what I was doing until my journal allowed me to spot it.

When I saw the pattern in my journal, I knew what I had to do. The first things to go were all the chemically laden detergents and supplies. It was amazing how much more space I had when I got rid of all the toxic cleaners. The duplication of products was amazing! Next, I organized my cluttered and chaotic laundry room so I could attack the dust, bacteria, and mold that had been gathering and growing there unmolested.

When I began organizing, I added a divided hamper to separate darks from lights and delicates from everyday items. (Since separating colors from whites meant having to do additional loads, which cost me more money and time, I always wished for a soap that would do that for me—in the wash. Being the little ol' soap maker, I came up with Soapworks Laundry Soap and Non-chlorine Bleach. It is so smart that it keeps your whites white and your brights bright all in the same load.) I made sure I had a clean, dust-free area to fold the clothes. No longer did I haul my clothes out of the laundry room and plop them on the floor where the dog had been. I used baskets to hold items that need extra attention.

Since this room represents only one thing—more work—we often neglect to clean it. How many people make it a regular habit to sweep, mop, and dust their laundry room? I have certainly been guilty of avoiding this habit. Mold, dust, mildew, and lint can be found in corners and under the washer and dryer.

Basement laundry rooms can be the worst because they have a tendency to be dark, damp, and unfriendly. That is a real incentive to do this cleaning chore, now isn't it? Laundry rooms in newer homes are often off the kitchen and are therefore more convenient, cleaner, brighter, and usually better maintained, which is as it should be.

My grandmother had her laundry room on the sunporch. For her, cleaning clothes was a sacred task that she did with love. Having this room be all windows and sunshine, a place where she could look out at her garden and rose bushes, made it a joy to be in, and it made doing laundry seem less like housework. Now I am not promising miracles here, but let's see what we can do to get the room cleaned up, not hazardous to your health, and not as bad a "honey do" chore as it might be.

# The Laundry Room Journal

In your journal, observe your clothes-cleaning habits. Do you prefer to do laundry every couple of days, or do you let it pile up and get it done in three of four loads at one time? Like some of you, I end up doing most of my laundry on the weekends. I made a promise to myself that I would change this habit and have begun doing small loads during the week so that I have more time with David on the weekends. Make sure when asking yourself about this room that you accommodate your habit, or, better yet, reexamine what will work best for you. Change may be what you need!

# Journal Questions: Laundry Room

### Questions to help locate toxins

1. Do I use laundry soap or detergent, and if so, how many products am I using to get the job done?

2. Do I store other household cleaners in this room? If so, how are they stored?

3. Are products such as outdoor bug and plant sprays and fertilizers in this room?

4. Is there dampness or mildew anywhere? Is there a damp, musky odor?

5. Are there any loose connections or wires in my washer or dryer?

6. Does anybody in the family become itchy after sleeping on or wearing freshly laundered linens and clothes? Do I get a rash around my bra or underwear? Do I react more when I'm hot?

7. Do I feel light-headed, nauseated, or out of sorts when doing the laundry?

### Questions to help organize

1. How many loads of laundry do I do per day/week/month?

2. Do I separate the clothes into easy-to-handle categories, such as special care items, dark, light, colored, and heavily stained clothes, and clothing that needs alterations?

3. Is everything I need available and within easy reach?

4. Can I get clothes out of the dryer, fold them, or quickly hang them up so I do not have to iron?

5. Is this area being used for other things than laundry; that is, is it a catchall for things that have no other home? If it is, is this the best area for these items?

6. Is doing the laundry easy, or is it something I dread? If I dread it, do I know why?

■  ■  ■

The following are the areas to consider in making the laundry room a healthier place to be:

■ organization

■ ventilation and air quality

■ products

■ cleaning

# Organization

In organizing the laundry room, your main focus should be to keep up with the inflow and outflow of clothes. This room should be organized with items such as shelving or cabinets for storing cleaning products, a table for folding clothes, something to hang clothes on to air-dry, and adequate space for laundry baskets to keep dirty clothes in until they can be washed. Poor room design as well as overcrowding with clutter or storage of other items can impede your goal of a healthy environment in the laundry room.

Invest in a laundry sorter and hanging racks so you can hang things up right from the dryer. This will save you lots of ironing time. Also, if you hang items when they're warm, you won't need to use other chemical products to take out the wrinkles. Using fewer products on them also extends the life of our clothes.

If you let things pile up, make sure you have big enough laundry baskets to hold the clothing so the clothes don't spill over onto the floor. This is really gross, especially in the basement. Floors equal bugs and more dirt, and if the clothes are at all damp, you're asking for a mess and a bad smell! Buy yourself an extra basket (or hanging hamper) and make sure the basket has holes in it to let air circulate, which will help prevent bacteria and mold growth. I suggest either a metal-framed hamper with porous bags or a wood-framed one with canvas bags. Please avoid plastic. It is another opportunity to cut down on the amount of outgassing in the house. Hampers with three separate bags for dividing colors are also nice.

Many times the laundry room becomes overflow storage for things that do not fit anywhere else. I have seen tools, an abundance of shoes, seasonal clothes, jackets, backpacks, and holiday decorations as well as toxic cleaners and paints kept there. Once again, you need to get into the "pitch and toss" mode, and if the laundry room is the only space available for the "leftovers," make sure the space is defined and separated from that for laundry items. This will limit confusion and definitely avoid accidents. See what is there and decide if it really should be there or if you need it at all. Often, the hot water tank is in this room. There should not be any toxic cleaners or flammable liquids nearby; this can be a fire hazard.

Part of keeping a well-organized laundry room is checking your appliances. A washer and dryer are a fact of life in most homes. It is only when one lets you down that you probably even consider what a great convenience they are. To keep these two appliances "healthy," check the connections that go from the washer and dryer to the wall. Make sure you have a seal (flat washer) on the inside of the female part of the hose that comes from the washer and goes to the water connection on the wall. There is also a small connector hose that can wear out over time. I recommend that every three months you peek behind your washer to make sure that that hose is still in good condition. (The washer costs 25 cents and the connector hose is less than $5, but the damage a broken one can cause can run into the thousands in damaged flooring.) If your hose breaks, damaged floors may not be the only problem; water damage can also create mold if not repaired and cleaned up properly. Remember, mold is a live entity and can easily move behind and up walls to infect other areas of your home. My advice is never try to clean up water damage on your own. Call in professionals to get the area dry as soon as possible. If it happens in the middle of the night, don't wait until morning to call a plumber. The long and short of it is this: If the seal looks even slightly old, replace it.

## Good, Better, Best:  **Organization**

**Good:**   Purchase a hamper that allows you to separate your clothes and also allows the clothes to breathe and not be "trapped."

**Better:**   Do not use the laundry room as a catchall for items that should be stored elsewhere. Color code your hamper or bag so that others can sort laundry as it gets placed in the hamper.

**Best:**   Check appliances regularly. Design the room for the laundry and define space for other items.

## Better Choice Mom Recommends

To get rid of odors in your washer, run a warm- or hot-water cycle with half a cup of baking soda. One cup of white vinegar once a month cleans out residue buildup in your machine and pipes. You can do these together or add more of one or the other, depending on which problem is greater. I do it monthly.

# Ventilation and Air Quality

In the laundry room, the dryer should vent outside. Sometimes the vent is directed indoors for humidification and energy savings, but this is not advisable, as odors and dust are circulated inside too. If you use toxic fabric cleaners or anticling chemicals (we will get to that no-no next) and have an inside vent, those chemicals are now releasing back into your home air. There are many side effects from heavy synthetic fragrances and the chemicals found in detergents, softeners, and anticling products, such as headaches, nausea, irritability and mood swings. I have a friend who used to say that doing the laundry made her sick. I would laugh because I thought she meant she just didn't like doing it—but she meant it really made her physically ill! In many homes, the laundry room does not get much air circulation, so the toxic cleaners release vapors that contribute to poor air quality. No wonder you feel lousy! If you have a window, let the sunshine in or at least crack a window.

Get rid of the chlorine bleach! This is particularly important for pregnant women and breast-feeding mothers. This cannot be stressed enough. If you must have the whitest of whites and don't want to switch to nonchlorine bleach, when your husband volunteers to help, turn him loose in the laundry. (You will also be glad you have the color-coded hamper!)

Mold and mildew in the laundry room can also contaminate the air. This is especially true for houses in which the laundry room is in the basement. It is common to have damp basements and leaks that have not been addressed. You should not have any damp areas in your house. Mold spores are released into the air and, like an infection, can penetrate into clothing or porous material. You can actually smell the mold on clothes that have been washed or stored in moldy basements. Believe it or not, people who have chronic problems get used to them and may not notice the smell. In that case, you can purchase mold test kits to check for contamination problems.

## Good, Better, Best:  **Ventilation and Air Quality**

**Good:**    Do the laundry with an open window and/or the vent on. Take a break for fresh air if you are doing multiple loads.

**Better:**    Clean the lint trap every time you do a load in the dryer.

**Best:**    Use all-natural laundry products that do not release toxins. Make sure the vent from the dryer releases outdoors and not back into the house. Create cross ventilation.

# *Products*

Toxic fabric softeners should be first on your list of items to get rid of and never use again. They are one of the most toxic products in the house and contain carcinogenic chemicals. They can cause damage to the lungs, brain, and nerves. The chemical residue saturates clothes and remains in the fabric for a long time. Fabric softeners often cause rashes and other skin irritations as well as systemic effects. The other hazard with fabric softeners is that toxic fumes are released when you run the dryer, which pollutes the outdoor air. Fabric softeners are totally synthetic, unnecessary, and toxic.

Some clothes that have been washed with fabric softeners will have to be thrown out because they are so saturated with chemicals. To get a clear idea of how toxic these softeners are, take a look at some of the specific ingredients and their side effects and cautions, as cited on the material safety data sheet for one of these popular grocery store products. Many individuals with multiple chemical sensitivities cannot even be in the same room with someone who has used a fabric softener on his or her clothes. We should be alert when sensitive individuals have such a reaction. The rest of us have become deadened to early warning signals, which means that we are able to poison ourselves without knowing it.

Some of the chemicals, and their side effects, in fabric softeners are the following:

- alpha-terpineol: aspiration into the lungs can produce pneumonitis or even fatal edema (swelling); irritating to mucous membranes; can also cause loss of muscular coordination.

- benzyl acetate: irritating to eyes and respiratory passages; do not flush to sewer; can be absorbed through the skin, causing systemic effects; carcinogenic (linked to pancreatic cancer).

- benzyl alcohol: irritating to the upper respiratory tract; can cause headache, nausea, vomiting, dizziness, drop in blood pressure, depression, and death in severe cases because of respiratory failure.

- chloroform: neurotoxic, anesthetic, carcinogenic; inhalation of vapors can cause headache, nausea, vomiting, dizziness, drowsiness, irritation of the respiratory tract, and loss of consciousness; chronic overexposure can aggravate disorders of the kidneys, liver, heart, or skin.

- ethyl acetate: may cause headache and narcosis, anemia with leukocytosis, and damage to the liver and kidneys.

- limonene: do not inhale vapor; irritant, sensitizer; prevent contact with skin or eyes; carcinogenic.

- pentane: harmful if inhaled; avoid breathing vapor; can cause headache, nausea, vomiting, dizziness, drowsiness, irritation of the respiratory tract, and loss of consciousness.

- Enough already!

There are natural alternatives to commercial fabric softeners. Borax is a great softener, deodorizer, and whitener. To use borax in your laundry, add half a cup to your wash. If you add half a cup of white vinegar to the rinse cycle, it will reduce static cling. To fight odors and soften clothes, add half a cup of baking soda. If you want your clothes smelling like something, add a few drops of essential oils to your wash cycle. Essential oils have the added advantage of having antiseptic properties. I dab a few drops of the oil onto my nightshirt or towel and throw it into the dryer with the load. This is so much better than fabric sheets. (Some essential oils will stain if you put them directly onto clothing, but adding a few drops to a tub full of water will not stain clothes.)

You should eliminate and replace synthetic detergents with soap-based products. Detergents are formulated from petrochemicals, and many contain bleaches, synthetic whiteners, and artificial fragrances. They were created to clean synthetic fibers but are not best for natural fibers like cotton, linen, silk, and wool. I quickly saw the difference between detergents and soap once I started making my own soap in my home and using the grated flakes diluted in water for cleaning clothes. I found that not only did my clothes come out cleaner, but they were 10 times softer than when I used a detergent. Doesn't the word "detergent" even sound rough? And rough it is on your skin and on your lungs. David's reaction to the harsh detergent chemicals was a huge, red hive-looking rash. You might experience subtle side effects yourself, such as headaches and nausea, from the residue on your clothes. If you wake up with headaches each morning, it may be your sheets. You just spent six to eight hours inhaling toxic fumes from your bedding. Now that brands of all-natural soaps are available in mass markets, I hope everyone stops using harsh detergents.

For bleach-o-philes, those interested in "whiter than white," try replacing your chlorine bleach with nonchlorine bleach products such as borax or baking soda. Stain removers and other mainstream toxic cleaners should be eliminated as well.

If you are fortunate enough to live in a warmer climate, hanging clothes outside is a great option, but only if no one in your family is allergic to pollen, which is in the air and will settle on your clothing.

This can definitely cause an allergic reaction. In warmer climates, the laundry room is often not air conditioned. You do not want to store your laundry soap or cleaning products in a room where the temperature gets too high; doing so will decrease the product shelf life. Natural products (you're switching to those now, right?) that contain ingredients such as essential oils may go rancid.

## Good, Better, Best: **Products**

**Good:** Reduce the number of toxic products. Rinse your washing machine with white vinegar to release dirt buildup so that it cleans more efficiently and you use less product.

**Better:** Double-rinse your clothing. Stop using bleach or softener—give up at least one. Use 100 percent natural essential oils if you want scented laundry.

**Best:** Get rid of all toxic, synthetic products and chlorine bleach. Buy natural cleaners: non-chlorine bleach and soap rather than detergent. Soften fabrics with baking soda or borax. For spots, use a nontoxic stain remover (see Suggested Readings for *Talking Dirty About Laundry* by Linda Cobb).

## Better Choice Mom Recommends

Try these nontoxic laundry aids:

- Soapworks: Liquid Laundry
- Soapworks: Powder Laundry
- Soapworks: Non-Chlorine Bleach
- Soapworks: Spot Remover
- baking soda to replace fabric softener
- White King: Laundry Booster (for whitening)
- Mule Team Borax
- Top of the Mountain Essential Oils

# *Cleaning*

Keep the laundry area clean. Do not let crust and crud build up in, under, or behind your washer and dryer. Bacteria, dust, and mold can build up and contaminate your clean clothes. If your laundry room is in the basement, you may need to install a dehumidifier to cut down on moisture and mold growth. Use natural products to clean the floor or other surfaces. Essential oils such as rosemary and lavender are naturally antiseptic and add pleasant fragrance.

The utility sink is an area of the laundry room that is often neglected and can be quite yucky. When was the last time you gave it a good, thorough cleaning? Usually this sink is for hand-washing items that are too delicate to place in the washing machine. It is also used to dye hair, rinse off tools, clean grease from dirty hands, and a variety of other activities. If you are going to have several different uses for this sink, make sure you clean it out after each use. You may even want to get a separate tub or bucket that you place inside the sink and use only for washing delicate clothing. Who wants to have her nylons or lingerie soaking in the same tub where Dad has just rinsed a paintbrush or leather protector for the car? If the sink is not thoroughly cleaned, toxins from those products can get onto your clothing.

By keeping the laundry room clean and organized, you support the purpose of this room: to clean your family's clothes safely and effectively.

## Good, Better, Best:  **Cleaning**

**Good:**    Don't bring in toxins to layer on toxins. Commit to no more than three toxic products in this room, if you must have any!

**Better:**    Purchase natural products. Clean behind the washer and dryer and under the sink regularly. Clean the lint trap on the dryer before every load. Check valves and seals to avoid more cleanup down the road.

**Best:**    Create boundaries for what gets cleaned in the laundry room and sink (no grease, tools, or cleaning of fish) or place a bowl in the sink to use for cleaning special items.

# *Better Choice Mom Wisdom*

For some strange reason, I now enjoy doing the laundry and find it relaxes me. No, I am not a nutcase. I love when all the laundry is done and put away. It may be because I get to see it go from huge, ugly mounds to neat, clean, well-organized piles. Now when I do laundry, I am not breathing in toxic fumes or getting toxic residue on my hands. Best of all, I'm returning to my son's dresser clean laundry that will not be harmful to him. Plus, I love being able to smell my son's natural scent and not the make-believe fragrance of "county fresh," whatever that is. He just smells like my son. I sleep much better at night knowing that there are no toxic chemicals on his clothes, sitting in his drawers, and hanging in his closet. I also like the peace of mind that comes with knowing that his sheets are clean and toxin free and that toxic residue won't interfere with his sleep.

Most of my friends, like many of you, perhaps, hate doing laundry. I am sorry to say, though, that laundry is something that is not going to go away. If someone figures out a way to make that happen, call me. To help yourself out, create as many tools as you can to make this chore easier and healthier. I went from doing laundry all day Sunday to doing it a few times a week or as needed. If there are other people in the home, perhaps having them help will be one of their weekly chores. Asking for help and having the family working together are positive things in creating a healthier home. I have had some great conversations with my son while the two of us folded laundry.

Though laundry may always be one of those "honey dos," there is no reason why you can't create an environment that you like as well as one that is healthy for you and your family. Oh, and one last question: Where do you think all those socks go?

# CHAPTER 10

# The Garage

## Out of Sight Is Not out of Mind

The greatest amount of wasted time is the time not getting started.
—Dawson Trotman

HOW EASY IT WAS for me to make mistakes and create a nightmare in my garage because, for me, the garage somehow was not part of my home. I thought it had no effect on us. Wrong! I stored many of David's things in the garage when they weren't in use, things like a baby stroller, car seat, and indoor swing. I forgot that while David's items were in the garage, they were absorbing toxins from paint, pesticides, plant fertilizer, and exhaust fumes. Even though I would clean them with nontoxic products before I stored them, I would just dust them off when I pulled them out. In almost no time, David was wheezing, his skin had broken out into a rash, and either he got glassy eyed or the "devil in my kid" syndrome would start.

I got the idea that the garage was not connected to me because when I was growing up, the garage was the domain of men. That is where my father and brother spent their time working on motorcycles, fixing cars, and taking on other macho projects in which I had no interest. I carried this mind-set into my adulthood, and my garage always felt like someone else's space. For me, the garage was a place to park the car and to store things. I thought little about it until one day I realized I could not get the car in there anymore, and I thought, What on earth happened?

Here is what happened: When I began to take the toxic things out of the house, create goals for each room in my home, and reorganize, all the discarded items were dumped into the garage, and I do mean dumped. Baby items got discarded for toddler's things, and then toddler's clothes and toys got discarded to make way for kids' things. The garage was filled with toys, clothing, swings, car seats, and strollers—all things that we tend to hold on to out of practicality or sentimentality. I can't get over how many car seats I went through as David grew. I had strollers in every style, from lay-down to sit-up, from umbrella to jogger strollers. All were in the garage, sitting in the dust, mold, oil, and gasoline and absorbing fumes from paint cans and car products.

In most homes, one of two approaches is used in the garage. Either things are perfectly organized with shelving, drawers, and hooks to hang things on—this was how my father's garage was, immaculate to the point that he even had everything labeled—or it is chaos, with overflowing boxes, displaced tools, garden equipment, old toys, holiday decorations, and a huge array of things people don't use but think they just might need one day. That was my garage.

If your garage is in the latter category and functions as a catchall room, you can change it with a little effort and education.

One of the biggest dangers in the garage is that we store some of our most toxic chemicals there. Gasoline, paints, strippers, glues, adhesives, and car cleaning products, to name a few, all have powerful and toxic ingredients. Just as in the bathroom or kitchen, storing these products together can be a hazard. And if your washer and dryer are in the garage, your clothes are absorbing these chemicals as well.

## *The Garage Journal*

It is time to take inventory. Take a look at what is lurking in the dark recesses of your garage. You might not feel that the garage is a priority because it's not "in the house." As I've just discussed, what's in the garage *can* affect the family's health and find its way into your home. Lack of time is the biggest reason for not being organized. Rolling up your sleeves and taking a look through your "I just couldn't throw it away" pile or "I am not sure, but I may need that" box gives you a boost and a sense of accomplishment. You may find treasures you forgot about or things that are long overdue to be thrown out. You may have a good laugh or a good cry. Either way, it can be cathartic physically, emotionally, or mentally, which is always a good thing. The best part? When you get organized and remove clutter, you are alleviating dust and places where mold might be an issue, discarding toxic products, and making the garage just as safe as any other part of your home.

## *Journal Questions: Garage*

### Questions to help locate toxins

1. When was the last time I really went through everything in the garage?

2. When was the garage thoroughly (and I mean thoroughly) cleaned?

3. What chemicals, heavy-duty cleaners, solvents, fuels, or other volatile products are stored here?

4. Do I really need these toxic products?

5. Am I aware of all the potential fire hazards in my garage?

6. Do I have flammable liquids stored near power tools, newspapers, or other materials that could cause a fire hazard? Can they be replaced with safer products?

7. How new is the car, and is it outgassing?

**Questions to help organize**

1. Do I buy items I may already have because I cannot find things in the garage?

2. Can I walk in and around the garage easily?

3. Can I get something out of the garage without things falling on me?

4. Am I comfortable with kids playing in the garage?

5. Is the garage safe?

■ ■ ■

The main concerns in the garage include the following:

- organization

- ventilation and air quality

- chemical hazards

# *Organization*

The organization of a garage varies greatly, depending on where you live. Since I was born and raised on the East Coast, our garage had to have space for snowblowers, tire chains, snow shovels, and an array of other equipment that pertained to the cold weather. People who live in the Southwest have no need for these items, but often what are stored in the garage are the kinds of things that are in the attic or basement of an East Coast home. No matter where you live, you need to adapt your garage to its use.

Although the garage's main purpose by design is storing vehicles safely, this often becomes secondary to other purposes. The second priority for the garage is usually to store many tools and electronics. Some garages have been made into a workshop. This is fine if you have things neatly organized. However, if the space is overcrowded and disorganized, it will interfere with your goal. Be clear about your purpose, and then make sure the garage environment actually matches this purpose.

Like many people, David and I store our bikes in the garage. Since riding his bike is a daily activity, it makes sense for him to have easy access. It is also important that closing the garage be easy for him so it doesn't get left open. After he had a few of his things taken from the garage, the message of closing the garage door got through to him loud and clear. But to make it really work for him, it had to be easy. Having David park his bike in the driveway, run around to the side of the house, go into the garage, hit the button, and run out (I am exhausted!) was way too complicated, and having him yell to me from outside to shut the garage door was way too annoying. I realized this system had to go. What I did was have the garage door company install a code box on the outside of the garage so that David could hop on his bike, hit a code, and then leave, making this entire process much easier on us both. Wish I would have done it sooner.

I also became concerned when I began to see David hanging out in the garage. It takes him a long time to get his bike, helmet, water bottle, and other items he feel he needs to go out to play. David is easily distracted and likes to look around and poke into stuff. Without thinking, I had stored many dangerous items well within his reach that could have had a devastating effect on him; I put them there because it was easier for *me* to reach them there. Paints, paint thinners, and gasoline all were stored on the ground by his bike. Seeing this made me realize that these items, too, needed to be in a safe place. The first thing I did was put my paint (just the colors that I still needed) in a locked cabinet.

The most common issue with the garage is overcrowding. Since this area can be the all-purpose storage room, it is easy to let the garage overflow with stuff. Usually, the longer you have been in your home, the worse it is.

It may be fairly easy to motivate yourself to clean out other areas of the home, but you may have trouble getting around to cleaning the garage. It can be more challenging than any one room in your house, so you avoid cleaning it.

If you're having trouble motivating yourself, I recommend that you read *Spiritual Housecleaning: Healing the Space Within by Beautifying the Space Around You,* by Kathryn L. Robyn (see Suggested Readings). She describes the process of sorting, purging, and reorganizing as therapeutic. By looking at the process from a different perspective, you may get inspired when you realize the deeper benefit you will achieve by doing the work. Then again, a pitcher of bloody Marys and some good tunes may be what does it! Whatever inspires you, get moving and do it.

I do suggest, though, that you try doing it little by little. Make it a goal to get rid of one box of "who knows what" every week. This can be an effective alternative to going in with great determination and then, after three hours of being up to your neck in "stuff," quitting. Not a good method.

I began to tackle the garage by first alerting the neighbors that I would be placing odds and ends in front of my house for a week or two. You don't want to upset the neighbors with your junk! Next, I rented a dumpster. Then, every day for two weeks, I set a timer for one hour and spent that time organizing my garage and laundry room (they are attached and are my storage rooms). After that, boy, did I get an attitude adjustment! It felt great having all that stuff gone, out of my life, finito!

My now-organized garage is a safe garage.

## Good, Better, Best: **Organization**

**Good:**   Lock away dangerous paints, thinners, and gasoline.

**Better:**   Take a look at what is in the garage and see what can be unloaded.

**Best:**   Set aside a weekend to organize, starting from top to bottom, and then keep it organized!

# Ventilation and Air Quality

The garage should have completely separate ventilation from the rest of the house. Ideally, the garage should not be attached to the house at all. Most people, like me, do not have a choice. If you are designing a new house or shopping for a new one, a detached garage is the "best" choice for health and safety. Otherwise, you want to minimize the amount of common wall between the house and the garage since, depending on the design and the insulation, the exhaust can seep into the home.

The worst choices are homes with the living quarters above the garage. The auto exhaust goes straight up into the house, where the people living there breathe it. Every time you start the car or drive into the garage, you are polluting the air in the home. You may have become used to the fumes or do not think it is a problem, but it is adding to the total load of chemicals that your body has to deal with. Individuals with multiple chemical sensitivities often have to park the car outside because they cannot tolerate the fumes. Vapors from chemicals such as paints or heavy-duty cleaners can also be contaminating the house from the garage.

The following are ways to cut down on air contamination from the garage:

- Seal any common walls with a nontoxic sealant, which can be purchased at any hardware store.

- Use a fireproof material on the garage side to create a barrier for fire safety as well as ventilation pollution. The barrier should already exist in the house since local fire codes require this as a safety measure; however, in practice this code is often violated.

- Do not operate any machines with combustion products in the garage for extended periods of time. That means cars, lawn mowers, snowblowers, or power tools. Make sure the garage door is open before and during operation to increase ventilation and reduce house contamination.

- Do not use harsh chemicals, volatile solvents, paints, fuels, or oils in the garage. If you have to use them, use them outside. Better yet, get rid of them altogether if they are not absolutely necessary.

- Make sure that there is no duct or opening that connects the garage area to the house. If there is, seal it off completely by redirecting the duct or vent or by blocking the open hole using proper building procedures.

- If you are highly sensitive to fumes, you can still park the car in the garage, but do not use the garage door to enter the house. Enter the house through the front door. In extreme cases, you can seal the door between the garage and the house to prevent air exchange and so it won't be used, which allows fumes to seep in every time the door is opened.

As for me, I don't want to take the chance of David inhaling any fumes from the car, so I back the car out of the garage, and David goes out the front door and meets me on the street. I also don't fill the car up with gas when David is with me; and I've instructed close friends and family to avoid doing that as well. Even with the windows rolled up, I don't want to take a risk. I also make him work on his bike or skateboard outdoors rather than sitting in the garage.

If your garage does contain a lot of toxic items, make sure to roll up the windows of your car when storing the car in the garage so you are not polluting the interior of the car. This is particularly important if you have a child seat in the car. As a resident of Phoenix, where garages get to be 120 degrees, I always have the windows open, so I have to be more cautious of what is in my garage.

## Good, Better, Best:  **Ventilation and Air Quality**

**Good:**   Open the garage door before you start the car. Pick up passengers on the street.

**Better:**   Make sure that any walls and vents common between the garage and the house are sealed. Do not enter the house from the garage, which allows fumes and exhaust to enter the house.

**Best:**   Have a garage that is detached from the house.

# Chemical Hazards

The garage can be a toxic melting pot.

## Paint

I can't believe how many less-than-half-full buckets of paint I had in my garage. People forget that paints have an expiration date. Very likely if you have old paint, it is thick, crusty, and no longer usable— time to get rid of it. Discarding of the gross paint cans (a few I could not even pry open) gave me much more space and alleviated the potential toxin hazard. (Note that paint requires special disposal because it's a toxic product.) For the paints I kept, I clearly labeled each can with the color and its manufacturer's number and brand and put a dab of the paint next to the number. No more mystery cans. When I finished using a can, I dabbed a sample of the color and wrote the brand and number on a board (one for inside and one for outside paint). When I needed to match the paint for repainting or touch-ups, I took the board to the paint store. This reduced the number of cans from "way too many" to two and completely eliminated the mystery can!

I also had many cleaners, most of which were half full. I told you I was a clean freak, but this was ridiculous. Many of the cleaners people store in their garage are toxic and outdated. Cleaners, if environmentally safe, should really be stored in the house. Until I really learned about chemicals, I had no idea how unsafe it is to store any kind of cleaning agents in areas where they are exposed to extremes of temperature (gee, just like in a garage). If you limit yourself to a few simple, safe products, there should be no need to have extra in the garage.

## Pesticides

Pesticides are designed to kill. They kill ants, fleas, mice, and roaches, among other creatures. According to the National Academy of Sciences, "suburban gardens and lawns receive heavier pesticide applications than most of our other land area in the United States," including agricultural areas. This is scary considering that most of us are not trained in how to safely use or store these products. Many people use them because they figure that since pesticides are legal, they must be "safe." They are absolutely not.

There is an alarming lack of research on how pesticides affect human health, and the toxicity information that does exist is not adequately communicated to consumers. Consider this:

- Studies suggest that pesticide exposure is linked to a number of health problems, including breast cancer, childhood cancer, and birth defects.

- Testing by the EPA is just beginning to look at long- and short-term health effects.

- Pesticides can be put on the market without complete health testing.

- Pesticide labels list "inert" ingredients, but this does not mean that these ingredients or chemicals are inactive. An EPA study of 1,200 inert ingredients found that 122 could cause cancer, birth defects, neurological disorders, or other health problems.

Pesticide labels are regulated by the Federal Insecticide, Fungicide and Rodenticide Act. Here are what the words on the labels mean:

- "Danger" (or "Poison," with skull and crossbones): could kill an adult if only a tiny pinch is ingested

- "Warning": could kill an adult if about a teaspoon is ingested

- "Caution": will not kill an adult until one ounce to one pint is ingested (Obviously, the damage would be far greater to a child.)

There are many ways to control pests naturally, and many times the natural way is much more effective. Some studies even claim that chemical pesticides are only creating stronger and more fit bugs! When you choose to use a toxic pesticide, you are also choosing to contaminate your own land, water, and air. Our choices have a ripple effect.

Another disturbing factor is that after we spray these products, they are on our clothes and shoes. We walk into the house, tracking those toxins onto rugs and floors. Heaven forbid you sit down on a stool in the kitchen for something to drink! (Remember in chapter

9 that I advised you to undress and put clothes in a laundry room and not in a hamper in the closet where you keep clean clothes? This is a perfect example of why I suggest it.)

## Fire Hazards

For those of us who have a water heater in the garage, many accidents happen here as well. The water heater contains an open flame, and when you store toxins, such as pesticides, paints, and lacquers that have fumes near the unit, the fumes can cause an explosion.

The following are more things to consider regarding fire hazards in the garage:

- Storing old newspapers, magazines, dirty rags, or boxes of clothes is not only unnecessary and unattractive but can also be a fire hazard, especially if they are stored near gasoline or other flammable liquids or a gas heater. Install a fire alarm and keep a fire extinguisher in the garage.

- The labels on most pesticides and toxic cleaners do not disclose their ingredients. They could be a fire hazard as well, and you would not even know it.

- Unplug power tools when not in use. If some power outlets are never used, put a plastic plug in them or, better yet, disable them completely. Shut them off at the circuit breaker if possible.

## Good, Better, Best: **Chemical Hazards**

**Good:** Do an inventory of toxic products and store them away from one another. Make sure there is a clear path around the water heater.

**Better:** Get rid of duplicate products, old cans of paint, and toxic pesticides and store any toxic products that you have determined are a must in a locked, fireproof trunk away from any heat source..

**Best:** Make your own natural fertilizer and pesticides. They work better!

# *Better Choice Mom Wisdom*

For years, I didn't care about the garage. After David's illness, I didn't have the luxury of thinking that way anymore. Every place David went into had to be as safe as possible. There was no purpose in clearing my home of toxins if one trip into the garage was opening my home to fumes through the air and if I was tracking toxins in on my shoes. As David gets older, where he goes is not as easy to control, so who knows what he will bring in. So, while he is home, I need to do my best to protect him.

With my garage now organized, I now know where my special dishes and appliances are, safely wrapped, still a part of my life, and available if needed. I love that the garage is now working with me and not against me. I feel good that I have space cleared around my water heater and that my paints are stored under lock and key. I love that David's area is defined so that where he stores his bike and skateboard is safe—no toxins or chemicals about.

By implementing the suggestions in this chapter, you'll reduce the possibility of poisoning, fire, and accidents. We all read about these tragedies and they hit home so many times because we are making the same mistakes in our lives. Be prepared and invest in the time to get rid of what you no longer need in your life—*move forward* by not letting old stuff hold you back. Improve your health by reducing the chemical exposure you may be getting from fumes that originate in the garage. Don't wait for an accident to happen. Making the garage a safer place can help you sleep better at night, knowing that you are making better choices—even in areas outside your comfort zone—for you and your family.

# Epilogue

Life is not a race, but a journey to be savored each step of the way.
—Anonymous

I HOPE YOU HAVE FOUND some valuable information in this book, but just as important, I hope you see that you can take back control of your life. My intent was to give you some ideas on how to take steps toward a healthier home and, in some small way, inspire you to take a look at your home in a different light. I think you can see from what I've shared of my journey that there are bumps, roadblocks, and crossroads. I cannot promise you a smooth trip. What I can tell you is that now that you are armed with greater knowledge and awareness, the obstacles will not appear to be as monumental as they once did. I hope I have given you the strength and courage to swim against the current and do what is best for you and your family.

I cannot stress enough to you that the greatest lesson I learned along the way was not to give my power away to anyone and not to let any situation make me feel helpless.

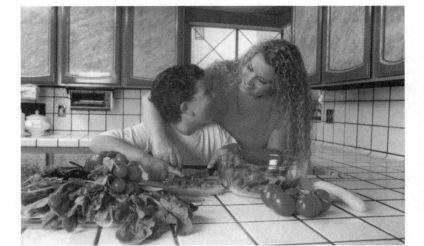

David and I enjoying each day.

I am here to tell you that you are most definitely not powerless or helpless! You know your children and your body better than anyone, so make that stand for something. If you don't believe that you can make changes and control your life, then no outsider or motivational book is going to make a difference in your life. Life's darkest moments are character building. They shape who we are and who we can become. I encourage you to embrace the challenges and dark moments. They move you to the light that much quicker.

Today David is a strong, active nine-year-old. He is playing football this year and just loves hanging with the guys! This summer I sent him to camp for the first year. He loved it, yet it broke my heart just a little that he could make it on his own for seven days without his mom. David will always have multiple chemical sensitivities. He will always have to be aware of his surroundings and avoid chemical exposures whenever possible. One of my biggest concerns while he was growing up was, "Will he be normal?" I can tell you that he is just like his friends—riding his bike through the neighborhood, having sleepovers, roughhousing with the dog—and I wouldn't have it any other way.

Finally, I am a mom, just like you. I take each day as a gift and try to live it to its fullest. That doesn't mean that there are not still times when I'm paralyzed with fear as I move into the unknown. But as I face and conquer challenges I once believed impossible, I grow stronger. As I've taken charge of my life, I've discovered a powerful woman inside me that I never knew existed. Find her within yourself; she is there.

# Appendix: Products, Services, Recipes

## General Suppliers

*The companies below carry a wide variety of safe household and personal care products, kitchen linens, filters, fabric, cushions, furniture, notions, beds, and bedding.*

Abundant Earth: (888) 513-2784,
    www.abundantearth.com
Janice Corp.: (800) 526-4237
Karen's Natural Products: (410) 378-4936
Living Source Catalog: (800) 662-878

## Specific Products

*The listings below are grouped by topic.*

### Air Duct Cleaning

National Air Duct Cleaners Association
    (NADCA)
1518 K Street, N.W., Suite 503
Washington, DC 20005
(202) 737-2926

### Baby Products, Bedding, and Nontoxic Toys

Baby Sleep Safe: www.babysleepsafe.com (product
    anchors crib sheets tightly)
Green Babies Organic: (800) 603-7508,
    www.greenbabies.com

Tiny Tush: (608) 356-2500, www.tinytush.com,
Wipes: (800) 987-6564, www.soapworks.com

Baby Bunz and Company
P.O. Box 113
Lynden, WA 98264
(800) 676-4559
    (diapers, baby and children's ware)

Dona Designs
825 Northlake Drive
Richardson, TX 75080
(214) 235-0485

Motherwear
P.O. Box 114
Northampton, MA 01061
(413) 586-3488

Pure Podunk, Inc.
Podunk Ridge Farm
R.R. 1, Box 69
Thetford Center, VT 05075
(800) 776-3865

Seventh Generation, Inc.
212 Buttery St., Ste. A
Burlington, VT 05401-5281

## Bedding

Heart of Vermont
131 South Main Street
Barre, VT 05641
(800) 639-4123

The Natural Choice
Eco Design Co.
1365 Rufina Circle
Santa Fe, NM 87501
(505) 438-3448
(800) 621-2591
    (Flooring, footwear, cleaning supplies, paints,
    filters, bathroom items)

## Building Supplies ("Green")

Building Health
102 Main St.
Carbondale, CO 81623
(800) 292(4838

## Candles

Britelites: (312) 957-0525, www.britelites.com

## Cleaning

Ecover Non-Chlorine Bleach: some local retailers
    or mail order
Murphy's Oil Soap: available at many retail stores
Oxi-Clean: many local retailers
Seventh Generation: (800) 456-1672,
    www.seventhgeneration.com
Soapworks Non-Chlorine Bleach: (800) 987-
    6564, www.soapworks.com

## EMF Information and Protective Products

EMF Safety Superstore: (518) 392-1946,
    www.lessemf.com
Field Management Service Corp.: www.fms-
    corp.com
Promolife.com: www.promolife.com
Shield to Protect: (760) 753-2121,
    www.emf-bioshield.com
Arronia AG (a German company):
    www.emf-meter.com

## Encasement Barrier Cloths

www.sneeze.com
Linens 'n Things: various brands of 100%
    untreated cotton

## Environmental Illness Information

American Academy of Environmental Medicine
    (AAEM)
4510 West 89th St.
Prairie Village, KS 66207
( 913) 642-6062; fax (913) 341-3625

## Essential Oils

Top of the Mountain Essential Oils: (800) 949-
    1884, www.thetopofthemountain.com
The National Association of Holistic
    Aromatherapy (an educational, nonprofit
    organization): www.naha.org

## Furniture

Bright Future Futon: (505) 268-9738
Heart of Vermont: (800) 639-4123
Pure Seasons: (800) 721-3909,
    www.pureseasons.com
Real Goods Trading: (800) 762-7325,
    www.realgoods.com
Shaker Workshops: (415) 669-7256

Simply Natural Home: (770) 794-0138,
www.simplynaturalhome.com
SOFA U Love: (310) 207-2540
Willsboro Wood Products: (800) 342-3373

## Home Accessories

*The following are stores that have a good selection of products to help you streamline your home. Be careful when purchasing because not all products will be all natural.*

Linens 'N Things: (866) 568-7378,
www.LNT.com
Bed, Bath & Beyond: (800) 462-3966,
www.bedbathandbeyond.com
Crate & Barrel: (800) 967-6696,
www.crateandbarrel.com
Cost Plus World Imports: (510) 893-7300,
www.costplus.com
Kitchen Classics: (602) 954-8141,
www.kitchenclassics.com
Pier 1 Imports: (800) 245-4594,
wwwpier1.com/home.asp

## Lightbulbs, Full-Spectrum

Light for Health, Your Source for Indoor
Sunshine: (800) 468-1104,
www.lightforhealth.com
Sun For Mood Full Spectrum Lighting: (888)
723-2852, www.sunformood.com
Full Spectrum Solutions: (888) 574-7014,
www.fullspectrumsolutions.com

## Laundry Products

Mule Team Borax: www.borax.com
Soapworks Liquid Laundry: (800) 987-6564,
www.soapworks.com
Soapworks Powder Laundry: (800) 987-6564,
www.soapworks.com
Soapworks Non-Chlorine Bleach:
(800) 987-6564, www.soapworks.com

Soapworks Spot Remover: (800) 987-6564,
www.soapworks.com
Top of the Mountain Essential Oils: (800) 949-
1884, www.topofthemountain.com
White King Laundry Booster (for whitening):
most retailers

## Mats for Children

Ayurveda Holistic Centers: (877) 989-6321,
www.ayurvedahc.com
GreenMarketPlace: (877) 989-6321,
www.greenmarketplace.com
YogaMats: (800) 720-YOGA (9642),
www.yogamats.com

## Oven and Window Cleaners

Soapworks All-Purpose Spray: (800) 987-6564,
www.soapworks.com
Seventh Generation brands of all-purpose
household cleaners
Bon Ami (scouring powder): most retailers

## Paint

Glidden Paints: ask your retailer for nontoxic
paint
AFM Enterprises: (619) 239-0321 (paint,
carpeting, flooring, wallpaper)

## Personal Care

Aubrey Organics personal care products: (800)
282-7394, www.aubreyorganics.com
Aveda personal care products: (866) 823-1425,
www.aveda.com
Bio Silk hair care products: (877) 701-1477,
www.jrussellsalons.com/biosilk.htm
Burt's Bees personal care and bath products: (919)
998-5200, www.burtsbees.com
California Baby bubble baths: (877) 576-2825,
www.californiababy.com
Eva's Esthetics: (800) 568-5886,
www.evaskincare.com

Paul Pender's products: www.paulpenders.com

Rocky Mountain sunscreen: (888) 356-8899, www.rmsunscreen.com

Salt Crystal underarm deodorant: many retailers

Soapworks bath wash and bars: (800) 987-6564, www.soapworks.com

Tom's of Maine personal care and dental care products: (800) FOR-TOMS, www.tomsofmaine.com

Zia skin care and body products: (800) 334-7546, www.zianatural.com

## Pest Control

Victor Poison Free and other pest control products: (914) 591-5516, www.victorpest.com, and many retailers

Orange Mate Citrus Spray: many retailers, such as Bed, Bath & Beyond and Linens 'n Things

## Safety Products for the Home

C. Crane Company: (800) 522-8863, www.ccrane.com

Comfort House: (800) 359-7701, www.comforthouse.com

Professional Equipment: (800) 334-9291, www.professionalequipment.com

Safety Hero, No More Hidden Dangers: (866) 626-SAFE (7233), www.safetyhero.com

## Sealants

Safe Coat: some retailers or paint stores, or order from the companies listed in General Suppliers in this appendix

Crystal Air: some retailers or paint stores, or order from the companies listed in General Suppliers in this appendix

## Toxin Testing

AccuChem: (214) 234-5412 (blood, urine, fat, and water testing)

Air Quality Sciences: www.aqs.com. (800) 789-0419 (chemical and microbial testing and tests kits)

Allergy Buyers Club.com Healthy Home Products & Information: (800) 789-0419, www.allergybuyersclub.com (formaldehyde tests for outgassing in furniture)

Anderson Laboratories: (800) 295-7344 (carpet and other household items testing; bioassay testing performed on rats)

Allerex
P.O. Box 239
Fate, TX 75132
(800) 447-1100

## Vacuums

Miele: www.miele-vacuum.com

Nilfisk: (800) 645-3475, www.pa.nilfisk-advance.com

## Wallpapers: Earth papers

Crown Corporation: some wallpaper retailers carry all-natural wallpaper from this company

Pallas Textiles: (414) 468-2600

# Recipes

## Cleaning

### Around the house tasks

Decal remover: soak in mixture of 1 part white vinegar to 1 part water; or spray mixture on decal and let sit until loose, and then gently scrape off.

Drain cleaner: mix half cup baking soda, half cup white vinegar, and 2 quarts boiling water.

Floor cleaner: mix 1 cup white vinegar and 2 gallons water.

Furniture polish: mix 1 tablespoon lemon oil in 1 pint mineral oil.

Furniture stain: dab on club soda and blot.

Pet odor remover: mix 1 part apple cider vinegar to 1 part water. Spray or dab on area and blot dry.

Rug/carpet cleaner: Dab on club soda. Or mix 2 parts cornmeal with 1 part borax. Sprinkle liberally, leave one hour, and vacuum. For tougher stains, blot repeatedly with white vinegar in soapy water.

Toilet bowl: make a paste of borax and lemon juice. To remove a toilet bowl water mark, apply toothpaste or rub with pumice stone.

Window cleaner: mix 2 tablespoons white vinegar in 1 quart warm water

Wood polish: mix 3 parts olive oil to 1 part white vinegar; or, for interior, unvarnished wood, try almond or olive oil

## Disinfectant spray

Combine 20 drops of a terpene essential oil (clove, cinnamon, rosemary, lavender) with 1 cup water in spray bottle.

## Stains

Food or juice stains: white wine vinegar takes out red food, soda, and juice stains.

Baby formula: dab lemon juice on the stain and lay out in the sun and then launder as normal; or make a paste of unseasoned meat tenderizer and water (3-to-1 ratio), rub on stain, let the paste dry, brush it off, rinse the fabric well, and then launder.

Blood: Soak washable fabric in a salt water solution. You may want to scrub lightly with an old toothbrush

Grass: use rubbing alcohol

## Washer/Dishwasher

To clean your appliance: add 1 cup white vinegar and $1/2$ cup baking soda (optional); run through a hot-water cycle without dishes or cloths.

## *Laundry*

Fabric softener: Pick favorite essential oil and dab on face cloth or sock and throw in dryer.

Wash: mix half to 1 cup baking soda and 3 to 5 drops natural essential oil

Anti-fungal and anti-bacterial: add cider vinegar and tea tree oil

Whitener: Use one part of 2 or 3 percent hydrogen peroxide to 8 parts water

Spot remover: Mix 1 part rubbing alcohol to 2 parts water in a clean spray bottle. Use as you would any other spot remover.

## *Personal Care*

### Bath Cookies

2 cups finely ground sea salt
$1/2$ cup baking soda
$1/2$ cup cornstarch
2 tablespoons light oil
1 teaspoon vitamin E oil
2 eggs
5 to 6 drops essential oil

Preheat oven to 350 degrees. Combine all ingredients to make dough. Shape into teaspoon-size balls and place on ungreased cookie sheet. (You can decorate cookies with clove buds, anise seeds, or dried citrus peel.) Bake cookies 10 minutes until lightly brown. Allow to cool. Drop 1 or 2 into bath and let dissolve. Makes about 24 cookies.

### Deodorant Powder

$1/2$ cup baking soda
$1/2$ cup cornstarch
Few drops essential oil (lavender, cinnamon, vanilla)

Place ingredients in glass jar; shake to blend. Apply with blusher brush.

## Liquid Deodorant

$1/4$ cup each witch hazel extract, aloe vera gel, mineral water

1 teaspoon vegetable glycerin

Combine in spray bottle. Makes about $3/4$ cup

## Hair Conditioner

$1/2$ cup honey

$1/4$ cup olive oil (use only 2 tablespoons for normal hair)

Combine. Work into hair. Cover hair with shower cap for 30 minutes. Rinse.

## Hair Gel

2 tablespoon flaxseed
1 cup water
An essential oil

Bring flaxseed and water to a boil. Set for $1/2$ hour. Strain when cool and drop in oil. Transfer to wide-mouth jar with lid.

## Sunblock

$2^{1}/2$ ounces sesame oil
$1^{1}/2$ ounces cocoa butter
$1/2$ ounce beeswax
4 ounces distilled water
2 tablespoons zinc oxide
25 drops grapefruit seed extract (a preservative)

Melt the oil, butter, and beeswax in double boiler over medium heat. Remove from heat, add water, and mix with electric hand mixer until thick and creamy. Add the zinc oxide and grapefruit seed extract. Store in glass jar with screw top. Makes 1 cup.

## Bugs

### Bug Repellant

1 teaspoon peppermint oil
1 teaspoon vegetable oil

Mix and dab on exposed skin with cotton ball.

### Fly Liquidator

1 pint milk
$1/4$ pound raw sugar
2 ounces ground pepper

Combine all ingredients in saucepan and simmer 8 to 10 minutes. Pour into shallow dish. Place out for flys. Flys attack it and soon will be suffocated.

### Fly Killer

1 egg yolk
1 tablespoon molasses
1 tablespoon black pepper

Mix together and set in saucer. Place on windowsill.

### Moth Repellant Sachet

2 ounces dried rosemary
2 ounces dried mint
1 ounce dried thyme
1 ounce dried ginseng
8 ounces whole cloves

Blend the herbs and place in natural sack. (Other plants for moth repellant are lavender, lemon, hyssop, winter savory, cedar shavings.)

# Web Sites and Links for Information

**Ammonia:** www.nsc.org/library/chemical/ammonia.htm

**Antibacterial cleaners:** www.nurseweek.com/features/98-10/soap.html and www.epa.gov/opp00001/kids/hometour/ products/disinf2.htm

**Borax:** www.borax.com

**Carcinogens:** www.physchem.ox.ac.uk/MSDS/carcinogens.html

**Chlorine:** www.mindfully.org/water/chlorine-water-miscarriages10feb02.htm

**Electromagnetic fields (EMFs):** www.dhs.ca.gov/ps/deoc/ehib

**Electrostatic filtration:** www.simplicityvac.com/buyer/features.html (link) or www.powertechindia.com/ele-fil.htm

**Environmental illness:** www.ourlittleplace.com/mcs.html

**Formaldehyde:** www.dhs.cahwnet.gov/ohb/HESIS/formal.htm

**HEPA:** www.hepa.com

**Material safety data sheets:** www.msdssearch.com

**Multiple chemical sensitivities (MCS) and Environmental Illness:** www.osha.gov.

**Negative-ion filtration:** www.wellnesstools.com/ionizers_more.pulp

**Ozonation:** www.osmonices.com/productspage844.htm

**Petroleum jelly:** www.physchem.ox.ac.uk/MSDS/PE/petroleum_jelly.html

**Seasonal affective disorder (SAD):**
www.discoveryhealth.com or www.umaine.edu/counseling/sigmund/sad.htm

**SIDS:** www.mercola.com/2001/jan/14/crib_death.htm.

**Volatile organic compounds (VOCs):**
www.doc.mmu.ac.uk/aric/eae/Air_Quality/Older/VOCs.html

# Suggested Readings

*Allergy-Free Living* by Dr. Peter Howarth and Anita Reid, Octopus Publishing Group Limited, London, 2000.

*Chemical Sensitivity* by William J. Rea, Lewis Publishers, 1992.

*A Consumer's Dictionary of Cosmetic Ingredients* by Ruth Winter, M.S., Crown, 1994.

*The Courage to Be Rich: Creating a Life of Material and Spiritual Abundance* by Suze Orman, Riverhead Books, 1999.

*Cross Currents: The Promise of Electromedicine, the Perils of Electropollution* by Robert Becker, M.D., Jeremy P. Tarcher, 1991.

*The E.I. Syndrome: An Rx for Environmental Illness* by Sherry A. Rogers, M.D., Prestige Publishers, 1988.

*Home Safe Home* by Debra Lynn Dadd. Jeremy P. Tarcher/Putnam Special Markets, 1997

*Is This Your Child? Discovering and Treating Unrecognized Allergies in Children and Adults* by Doris J. Rapp, M.D. (Doris J. Rapp, M.D., F.A.A.A., F.A.A.P., is a board-certified environmental specialist and pediatric allergist and founder of the Environmental Research Foundation, P.O. Box 60, Buffalo, NY 14223; (800) 787-8780), William Morrow, 1992.

*Is This Your Child's World?: How You Can Fix the Schools and Homes That Are Making Your Children Sick* by Doris J. Rapp, Bantam Doubleday Dell, 1996.

*Light Medicine of the Future* by Jacob Liberman, O.D., Ph.D., Bear & Co., 1992.

*Living Without Magazine*, P.O. Box 2126, Northbrook, IL 60065; www.Living Without.com: see "Water Wisdom: In the Know About H20," summer 2001.

*Love Is in the Earth: A Kaleidoscope of Crystals* by Melody R. R. Jackson, Earth Love Publishing House, 1995.

*A Natural Guide to Pregnancy and Post Partum Health* by Dean Raffelock D.C., Robert Rontree, M.D., and Virginia Hopkins with Melissa Block, Avery, 2002.

*Nine Steps to Financial Freedom: Practical and Spiritual Steps So You Can Stop Worrying* by Suze Orman, Three Rivers Press, 2000.

*The Nontoxic Home and Office* by Debra Lynn Dadd, Jeremy P. Tarcher, 1992.

*Nontoxic, Natural and Earthwise: How to Protect Yourself and Your Family from Harmful Products and Live in Harmony with the Earth* by Debra Lynn Dadd, Judy Collings, and Steve Lett, Jeremy P. Tarcher/Putnam Publishing Group, 1990.

*The Poisoning of Our Homes and Workplaces: The Truth about the Indoor Formaldehyde Crisis* by Jack Trasher, Ph.D., and Alan Broughton, M.D., Seadora, Inc., 1989.

*The Sick Building Syndrome* by Nicholas Tate, New Horizon Press, 1994.

*Spiritual Housecleaning: Cleaning the Space Within by Beautifying the Space Around You* by Kathryn L. Robyn, New Harbinger, 2001.

*Talking Dirty About Laundry* by Linda Cobb, Pocket Books, 2001.

*Talking Dirty with the Queen of Clean* by Linda Cobb, Pocket Books, 2000.

*Toxic Carpet* by Glenn Beebe, A O P R, Incorporated, 1991.

*Trade Secrets* (PBS documentary) by Bill Moyers, www.pbs.org/tradesecrets. This recent documentary claims a pattern of cover-ups by the vinyl chloride industry of workers getting sick and dying from exposure. The show brought swift response from the industry, claiming Moyers omitted key facts. Access the industry response at www.abouttradesecrets.org.

*Your Home Health and Well Being* by David Rousseau, W. J. Read, M.D., and Jean Enwright, Hartley & Marks, 1998.

# Index